The International Library of Psychology

THE PSYCHOLOGY OF TIME

T0174043

Founded by C. K. Ogden

The International Library of Psychology

GENERAL PSYCHOLOGY
In 38 Volumes

THE PSYCHOLOGY OF TIME

MARY STURT

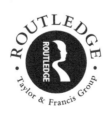

First published in 1925 by
Kegan Paul, Trench, Trubner & Co., Ltd.

Reprinted in 1999, 2001 by
Routledge

2 Park Square, Milton Park, Abingdon, Oxfordshire OX14 4RN

711 Third Avenue, New York, NY 10017

First issued in paperback 2014

Routledge is an imprint of the Taylor and Francis Group, an informa business

Transferred to Digital Printing 2006

British Library Cataloguing in Publication Data
A CIP catalogue record for this book
is available from the British Library

The Psychology of Time
ISBN 978-0-415-21041-6 (hbk)
ISBN 978-0-415-75806-2 (pbk)
General Psychology: 38 Volumes
ISBN 978-0-415-21129-1
The International Library of Psychology: 204 Volumes
ISBN 978-0-415-19132-6

PREFACE

" THE psychologist may if he pleases make the gradual development of our ideas of time the object of his inquiry, though, beyond some obvious considerations which lead to nothing, there is no hope of his arriving at any important result." Lotze, *Metaphysic*, B. II, ch. iii.

This harsh prediction is perhaps not entirely without justification to-day. By itself any subject—even metaphysics—is largely helpless before the study of Time. Time lies on the confines of so many subjects : anthropology, astronomy, metaphysics, theology, physics, mechanics, mathematics, logic, and psychology, and even the poets have something to say about it. I have attempted to put together a sketch of the subject keeping these different aspects in mind, even if I have not treated of them directly. I could not have treated of any one of them except in outline in a book of this size, and my lack of specialist knowledge has saved me from attempting an encyclopædia. The book is psychological in that the point of view throughout has been dictated by human experience. There is theory, but it is based on observation and sometimes on experiment. If the experiments seem crude I must plead necessity. The facilities for psychological research in this country are so inadequate that I have had to do the work out of touch with a laboratory, with apparatus but a stop-watch. I have, however, lamented the necessity less in this subject than I should have done in others, because it seems to me important, in dealing with time, to preserve an air of reality, and the ordinary person has little appreciation of periods less than $\frac{1}{5}$ of a second, and these are shown on an ordinary stop watch.

Part of this book has already appeared in the British Journal of Psychology and in the Report of the Psychological Congress held at Oxford in 1923. I must thank Dr. Myers for his kind permission to use this material again here. I also offer my thanks to Dr. Curzon for reading the MS. and for many very helpful criticisms.

J. C. Oakden has saved me from many mistakes in mathematics. I am very grateful, and if there are any mistakes left it is my fault.

Lastly, I must thank my subjects, and one in particular, for submitting on so many occasions to being bored.

Nil ego contulerim jucundo sanus amico.

M. S.

CONTENTS

CHAPTER I

THE METAPHYSICAL VIEW OF TIME

FEW subjects have received more attention and advanced less than a study of the nature of time. It is a subject to which metaphysicians, psychologists, mathematicians, and physicists have approximately equal claims, and to it, at one time or another, all have devoted themselves. Approached from such different standpoints the subject ought to have been rapidly explored. Instead of this, the various investigators have hampered or ignored each other. The metaphysicians have written without regard to psychological findings, and ended by a mutual confutation. The mathematicians have evolved such views of time as have been forced upon them by the physicists, with the result that their conception of time has been turned topsy-turvy within recent years; and that, just at the moment when metaphysicians were getting well used to Newtonian time. The psychologists, with a few brilliant exceptions, have devoted endless time and a perfected experimental technique to the elucidation of points so minute, and pursued under conditions so artificially simple, that the ordinary man is quite at a loss to see what relation such work bears to common experience. The result naturally has been that psychological views of time have had little influence on metaphysics or science; and, when psychological findings are utilized, it is rather those of thirty years ago than more recent discoveries.

B

This book is an attempt to bring together, however inadequately, some of the knowledge about time which has a psychological bearing, and for this purpose it has been necessary to adopt a definite view as to the nature of time. No psychologist can accept time as something objectively real and unchanging, since such a view reduces the experiencing mind to a mere observer, and the variations which are so noticeable a feature of the time-experience become just so many errors and failures in observation. Merely to catalogue the mind's lapses is a dispiriting task. The natural assumption to make is that time is a concept which is built up through individual and racial experience. It is then possible to trace the development of this concept and to note the different forms it takes under different conditions. Divergences from the normal are not errors, but rather curious adaptations to special circumstances. This involves the further assumption that time is subjective, i.e. that it is created by our own minds, and is not something objectively existing like a table, nor is it a quality of objects such as a colour. It may be necessary to say a few words in defence of this assumption.

Early in philosophical thought it was realized that time did not possess the material reality of e.g. a table. Aristotle and Zeno the Stoic, both make time non-material. Aristotle defines time as ἀριθμὸς κινήσεως κατὰ τὸ πρότερον καὶ ὕστερον,[1] and Zeno says χρόνος ἐστι κινήσεως διάστημα.[2] This view has not seriously changed (in spite of the fact that most languages possess a concrete or proper noun for time), and most people, like Alice, speak of time as "it"

[1] *Phys.* iv, 11, 219, b. 2.   [2] *Fragments.*

and not " he ", and would be greatly surprised if time manifested a material existence either by affecting any of the special senses, or by producing any other definite changes ascribable to it alone.

However, to deny time a material existence does not mean to deny it objective existence altogether. It may be a quality of things as a colour or motion is, or it may have an all-pervasive existence such as the ether of space was once assumed to possess. The Greek quotations suggest that time was at one period considered to possess an existence very similar to that of motion. Even when the question of how we apprehend time had been raised, there was little sign that time itself was regarded as unreal. This is well illustrated by Locke's attitude in the *Essay*. The psychological observation is exact, but there is no hint. that we are creating time, and not simply apprehending it. " Our measures of duration cannot any of them be demonstrated to be exact. Since no two portions of succession can be bought together, it is impossible ever certainly to know their equality. All that we can do for a measure of time is to take such as have continual successive appearances at seemingly equidistant periods ; of which seeming equality we have no other measure but such as the train of our own ideas have lodged in our memories, with the concurrence of other probable reasons, to persuade us of their equality." [1] And though he is quite awake to the variations in the estimate of time which frequently occur, Locke holds that, on the whole, our judgment of time is very fairly in accordance with reality. Since our ideas

[1] *Essay*, bk. ii, ch. xiv, § 23.

" whilst we are awake succeed one another in our minds
at certain distances not much unlike the images in the
inside of a lanthorn turned round by the heat of a candle.
This appearance of theirs in train, though, perhaps it may
be sometimes faster and sometimes slower, yet, I guess,
varies not very much in a waking man ".[1]

The most definite assertion of the objectivity of time
was made by Newton in the interests of mathematics.
Previous to Newton, the relation of time to mechanics and
astronomy had been very inadequately perceived.   For
example, it was only in his day that the ideas of force and
time were connected and that geometry and chronometry
in astronomy were found to be dependent on each other.
Even in Newton's own laws of motion the time factor is
rather implied than expressed.   He writes : " Change of
motion is proportional to the impressed force," when what
is really meant is that the " *Rate* of change is proportional
. . ." the rate of change being reckoned according to a
graduated scale of *time*.   It was therefore necessary to stress
the time element in mathematics, and the science of his
day was best served by a time which " in itself and from its
own nature flows equally " and which was capable of
infinite subdivision.

So definite an assertion naturally provoked criticism.
Berkeley, starting from the succession of our ideas, saw in
this succession the very essence of time, not " only the sensible
measure thereof " ; and he declared that if he went farther, he
was plunged into a sea of difficulties and confusion.   " For
my own part, whenever I attempt to frame a simple idea of

[1] Ibid. § 9.

time, abstracted from the succession of ideas in my mind, which flows uniformly and is participated in by all beings, I am lost and embrangled in inextricable difficulties. I have no notion of it at all." [1]

The reason for this was partly the impossibility of imagining what " empty time " would be like, partly the logical difficulties of a time which is infinitely divisible and discrete. " I have no notion of time at all," reiterates Berkeley, " only I hear others say that it is infinitely divisible, and speak of it in such a manner as leads me to harbour odd thoughts of my existence ; since that doctrine lays one under an absolute necessity of thinking either that he passes away innumerable ages without a thought, or else that he is annihilated every moment of his life, both which seem equally absurd."

Berkeley is not alone in his difficulties ; even those who would uphold the existence of time find it difficult to give any satisfactory account of its manner of passing.

Mr. F. H. Bradley, in one of his earlier books, has given us a picturesque account of time. " We seem to think that we sit in a boat and are carried down the stream of time, and that on the bank there is a row of houses with numbers on the doors. And we get out of the boat and knock at the door of No. 19, and, re-entering the boat, then suddenly find ourselves opposite 20, and having there done the same, we go on to 21. And, all this while, the firm fixed row of the past and future stretches in a block behind us and before us. If it is really necessary to have some image, perhaps the following may save us from worse. Let us fancy ourselves

---

[1] Principles, § 98.

in total darkness, hung over a stream, and looking down on it. The stream has no banks, and its current is covered and filled continuously with moving things. Right under our faces is a bright illuminated spot on the water, which ceaselessly widens and narrows its area and shows us what passes away on the current, and this spot that is light is our now, our present." [1]

It may have been the improbability of this picture of time that influenced him, but at any rate in his later work Mr. Bradley denies the reality of time and definitely condemns it as Appearance. Our ideas of time are hopelessly self-contradictory, and therefore time can have no real existence. " If we take time as a relation between units without duration, then the whole time has no duration, and is not time at all. But, if you give duration to the whole time, then at once the units themselves are found to possess it, and they thus cease to be units. Time, in fact, is 'before' and 'after' in one ; and without this diversity it is not time. But these differences cannot be asserted of the unity, and on the other hand, and failing that, time is helplessly dissolved." [2] A few pages on he continues the argument. " If we take the presented time, that involves change, a ' now ' becoming a ' then '. Thus, if in any time we call presented there exists any lapse, that time is torn by a dilemma, and is condemned to be appearance. But if the present is timeless another destruction awaits us. Time will be the relation of the present to a future and a past ; and this relation, as we have seen, is not compatible with diversity or unity." [3]

[1] F. H. Bradley, *Principles of Logic* (1883), p. 53.
[2] F. H. Bradley, *Appearance and Reality*, p. 39.
[3] Ibid.

It is possible to meet a logician on his own ground, and argue for the necessity of time ; but far more serious for the Newtonian view of time is the defection of the scientists for whose benefit it was invented. The modern theories of relativity have destroyed Newtonian time theoretically, but they offer time a continued objective existence as a fourth element in a space-time continuum. This theory of time is prompted, as was its predecessor, by mathematical and physical considerations. For the adequate determination of any event four co-ordinates are necessary, the three provided by space and the fourth by time ; and time is, therefore, treated as being real and as corresponding to space. This reality, however, is not incompatible with variations due to particular circumstances. For an observer on a moving platform, time is different from what it is for a stationary observer. Time is thus not unitary, but individual, and differs according to the circumstances in each particular case. It can also be imagined to differ on a larger scale, according to the different types of curvatures which space-time may possess.

Such a theory opens fascinating fields for the psychologist, and it is noticeable that psychological considerations are not infrequently appealed to in discussions of this subject, though this appeal is generally rather half-hearted.[1] Actually, of course, if the theory were anything but a hypothesis of the scientists, the decision as to the nature of time would lie with psychology, and time would *be* such as it might appear on investigation to seem to be. There is, however, little likelihood of such an appeal being made ; time will

[1] Broad, *Scientific Thought*, p. 463, and elsewhere.

have its nature decided in accordance with the necessities of physics and mathematics, and when these necessities change so will time.

Lastly, time can hardly be a quality of things as colour is. If it is a quality it belongs, or can belong, to all things equally, and only affects us in an indirect way. We have no sense for time as we have for taste or smell or surface texture. We cannot perceive it directly. We do perceive that things change, and this perception of change is our nearest approach to a perception of time. It has often been maintained that to deny the objective existence of time is to deny the possibility of change, but if we admit change we are not therefore forced to admit the existence of time, at least as an objectively real entity. Time and change are doubtless closely connected, and much of what we mean by time involves change, but our concept of time is more than change. It includes a future, a past, and a scheme of organization. We may know that a thing has changed because in its presence we have a feeling of unfamiliarity. This *may* imply a reference to the past, but this reference is extremely slight, and may even be lacking altogether. The feeling of the past is, as has often been pointed out, a present feeling, and it is quite possible to imagine a being possessed of so rudimentary a memory that a feeling of familiarity did not call up any image of a previous state of things. We cannot then be forced to admit that time, as we know it, is real even if we regard time simply as the precondition of change ; and, moreover, time has apparently too definite qualities of its own to be treated in that way. Besides, time which is merely the condition of change, is not satisfactory for any of the purposes either of the mathematician or the psychologist.

If time is not objective, it must be subjective, and due to our own minds. The most famous exposition of this view is of course Kant's. Time for Kant is not given by external objects, but is the form under which we apprehend phenomena. It is . . . " nothing else but the form of the inner sense, that is, of the perception of ourselves and of our inner state. For time can be no determination of external phenomena." [1]

" If we abstract from the manner in which we immediately perceive our own inner state, and mediately all external phenomena, and think of objects in themselves, we find that in relation to them time is nothing at all. Time is therefore a purely subjective condition of human perception, and in itself, or apart from the subject, it is nothing at all." [2]

This view raises two problems, the psychological question " How do we come by this concept of time ? " and the metaphysical, " Are time and change foreign to the real nature of things ? " The first question is of importance here, the second can be left aside as having no immediate psychological bearing. Kant maintains that the concept of time is, as it were, ready made in our minds, and is not derived from experience, but applied to it, being indeed a " pure form and the a priori condition of external phenomena ".[3]

This decision has naturally been disputed. It is hard to

---

[1] Kant, *Transcendental Aesthetic*, § 2, 6 (b).
[2] Ibid. (c).   [3] Ibid.

have the origin of such a fascinating thing as the sense of time wrapt in dark clouds of a-priority and mystery. Time is as fair a psychological game as any other. In consequence, Spencer, Guyau, James and the writers of many textbooks have all rushed in where Kant refused to tread.

Time cannot be a-priori in the Kantian sense, because the knowledge of it both develops in the individual and appears to vary in different cases. It is possible to discover within the limits of human experience great differences in the power to apprehend time and to deal with temporal ideas. This power seems to vary partly with the age of the individual and partly with the degree of culture of the people concerned. It is also possible to find within the experience of an educated adult great differences of time experience on different occasions. There is even very little reason, except for a sentiment for philosophic tidiness, to believe that the times of various people are the same, or that any one person has a completely unified time. The relativists have gone a long distance in this direction, but they still appear to cling to an absolute super-personal time based on the velocity of light. The practical man believes in a single time because he is able to co-operate in matters of time with others, catch his train, and keep his appointments ; but, theoretically, this comparative synchronization, assisted as it is by artificial means, does not disprove the possibility of many individual times, once time is admitted to be subjective and not objective.

There is, therefore, no good reason for refusing to believe that time is a concept that is built up in the course of the life of the individual and the race. Whether it is a satisfactory concept depends on the use to which it is put. It is quite possible to prove, as have Kant and Bradley, that it is inconsistent and rent asunder by contradictions ; but to do so it is necessary to transfer the concept to a sphere of thought for which it was never intended. The needs of life, and the ordinary experience of mankind, do not involve us in difficulties over the infinite divisibility of time,[1] nor its infinite extension. We do know very short periods of time ; but when two clicks are separate by a sufficiently short period, i.e. about $\frac{1}{100}$ second, they are perceived as one, and *for us* time can be no further subdivided. In the same way, we experience long periods of time and imagine longer ; but with eternity we have nothing to do—at least not in this existence ; our ideas concerning it are necessarily vague and liable to be confused. It is not uninteresting to consider the form that such ideas take in men's minds, but the failure of these ideas to stand metaphysical criticism does not invalidate them or render them useless within their own sphere. This book will therefore assume that time is a concept, and a good concept for its own purposes, but will end with a short discussion of the psychological theory of the nature of time, and the possible anomalous " times " that may be invented or experienced.

[1] The Quantum Theory may do so, but so far it is confined to times with which only the scientist can deal.

CHAPTER II

ORIGIN OF TIME EXPERIENCE

THE earliest forms of time experience are naturally not matters for direct experiment or observation. They belong to stages of development or to forms of life concerning which we can form little else but guesses and hypotheses. The telling of psychological fairy tales has a certain attraction, but it would be unwise to attribute to an account of the experience of a crab any high degree of scientific validity. With this proviso I will commence this chapter.

Within that experience which may be called temporal, various elements can be distinguished. Writers such as Spencer, Kant, and even Locke, are too apt to speak as if the time experience consisted of nothing but the perception of the succession of our ideas, and as if the whole problem was how we came to think of time as passing in a stream. This serial order of time is important and bulks largely in the time experience of the adult, but it is far from primitive, and an attempt to confine a discussion of time to this aspect of the experience results in omitting a consideration of some of the most interesting points connected with it.

The time experiences which appear to be primitive are (a) the apprehension of an event as having duration in time, and as being temporally extended in the same manner as a contact may be spatially extended.

(b) The apprehension that an event has occurred before, or that one event has occurred before, or will occur after, another. From this arises the concept of the past, and later of the future.

(c) The experience of two things occurring simultaneously. In its simplest form this experience occurs when the two events affect the same sense organ ; in a more complicated form they affect different sense organs.

These three elementary experiences must be very different in their simplest form from anything which we can know, because, in our case, they are overlaid by a great deal of experience which is far from primitive and due to the inclusion in our time of elements arising from late constructions.

For us, events are arranged in relation to a conscious subject with a history and future of its own. However little we may intentionally relate events to ourselves, we always do connect each new event with our past as part of one life history. In this way no time moment comes to us disconnected, but always in relation to a past or future which has more or less definite characteristics. Moreover, this life history is for each of us single. An event learned through sight is apprehended as before or after, in a single time, an event learned through touch. I see my kitten sitting on the floor. I stroke it, it moves, and I stroke it again. The sights and touches are apprehended as belonging to a single time history. There is not one series of touches and another of sights.

Secondly, when we think of time, we think in terms of a conventional time which possesses units. We think of hours, days, minutes, and we think of each of these units as always being of the same length. The more experience we have, the more facility we get in the accurate use of these units, and the smaller units we can use. These units, which are qualitatively alike, are distinguished by numbers, and, theoretically, each second that passes is fully distinguished from any other by number. We do not, however, generally think in such short units as seconds or distinguish them from each other ; but we do habitually so distinguish days and perhaps hours.

Going further, we think of the world as possessing a history like an individual, and we relate events to this world history in the same way that we relate them to our own, giving them absolute position in a single time order.

Lastly, we abstract the particular events which occupy the different instants of time and conceive of an abstract entity Time which can be divided into present, past, and future, and which " flows " according to certain laws.

These different additions to the primitive time experience will be spoken of in different places. In this chapter the primitive experience and the first stages of organization into a single time will be discussed.

In the earliest stages none of these later elements need be involved. We could have all our three primitive time experiences without the addition of these four later ones ; but the primitive experiences would be very different from anything which we ourselves know. How different they would be can be realized from an attempt to represent this primitive time experience in isolation from the later additions.

For us, duration involves the question " how long " and
a reference to a conventional time scheme, but there is no
necessity for it to do this. In our own experience it is not
uncommon to lose all sense of the conventional measurement of time, and, at a period when time measurements
were less exact and less common, this must have been of
more frequent occurrence. In a simple organism the
experience of continued existence, or of continued stimula-
tion, need have no reference to anything beyond itself ;
nor need the durations of different periods be compared
with each other or with any conventional series. In a
similar way the experience of succession does not necessarily involve the arrangements of events in a time line.
To know that something has occurred " before " only
relates that event to the present, not to other events in the
past. Nor again is it necessary to postulate a unitary time
experience for lowly forms of life. Fouillée, in his introduction to Guyau's *Genèse de l'Idée de Temps*, suggests
that sequences of events coming from different sense organs
were not at first synthesized into a single unitary time. An
animal might have several " times " ; the " time ", or
succession of events, of vision must have been different
from that of touch, and it was only with later developments
that these were synthesized, so that the creature discovered
that *after* the sight of a rock he touched it.

The speculation is interesting, and is supported by a
certain difficulty that can be found among men in deciding
on the simultaneity or successiveness of impressions. When
separated by a certain time interval (10-20σ) touch and
sound stimuli are judged simultaneous ; at a longer

interval (30-40σ) they are definitely successive ; but at an intermediate interval (20-30σ) the subject finds it extremely hard to judge whether they are simultaneous or not, and to decide in which order they occurred. This difficulty may indicate that the power to synthesize into *one* time order experiences coming from different senses has been acquired in the course of evolution, and, though fairly efficient in us, is not completely so.

Lastly, even the judgment of rate of movement need not involve any conscious calculation or comparison. The cat who jumps and catches a running mouse, the tennis player who hits a moving ball, and the " stroke " of an eight who increases the rate of his stroke by so many a minute are stages in the development of this judgment which, as we know from our own experience, in no way depends for its success on calculation.

The time experience, then, of a very simple creature must be extremely vague. There must be the rudiments of the experience of duration—a certain temporal extensity of experience, there must be an experience of the familiarity or strangeness of certain events ; a recurrent hunger or satiety ; and the perception of stimuli coming from different senses. From these largely non-temporal elements the concepts of past, present, and simultaneity develop, and the whole elaborate superstructure of conventional time is built up.

This development is only one aspect of the increasing complexity of the organism and its more exact adjustment to the different circumstances of life. If it is considered here as being largely due to the increased powers of memory and purpose, these words must be taken in a wide sense as indicating the general retentiveness of the organism, and the gradually increasing consciousness of its instinctive aims.

We can take in turn the different elements in the primitive time experience and show in outline how they might have developed. A creature absolutely without memory would be unable to apprehend any duration beyond, possibly, the shortest. What this would be for so lowly an animal as the sea-anemone it is impossible to guess, but in man there appears to be a duration which can be apprehended " intuitively " (anschaulich) as a whole. If memory were abolished we should be unable to apprehend any period longer than this, and it appears to be about 550σ.[1] Lower in the animal scale deficiencies of memory must reduce the length of a period that can be apprehended as such to the duration of this specious present, and the increase of the period which can be experienced as a unit must depend on a combination of memory with the power of steady attention. This attention, in turn, is one aspect of the organization of purpose and takes its origin from it. A creature low in the scale, or a human child, usually does not show any great concentration of attention or stability of purpose ; in this stage the activities which are long continued, as when a sea-anemone waves its tentacles for hours at a stretch, are not actions which necessarily involve any definitely co-ordinated activity, nor is one part of the action definitely influenced by the preceding parts. There

---

[1] Cf. W. James on this " specious present " : *Principles of Psychology*, ch. xv, and Myers, *Text-book of Experimental Psychology*, ch. xxiii.

is no apparent reason why the period of an anemone's tentacle waving should be organized into a " period " of time in the way that a dog's rabbit-hunting might form a period. In the latter case actions succeed one another in an order determined by the changing conditions under which the end is perused ; in the former the activity is not thus guided from stage to stage, and an anemone, by forgetting previous actions, would not impair the efficiency of the present one.

Further developments of the experience of duration are also largely dependent on memory, though in many cases the memory images are not made explicit. In particular, this is the case in estimating rate of movement. Skill in any occupation involving movement has to be learnt, and the way in which it is learnt can conveniently be studied by watching a kitten practising with a cotton-reel. The kitten's progress in achievement depends partly on increasing muscular development, but also on an actual knowledge of relative rates of movement of itself and the reel. This comparative judgment of time has extraordinary developments when we come to time measurements by clocks or swinging pendulums. In the primitive form of this judgment we adjust our own actions to the movements of some other moving body, in the developed form we correlate our own activity with the movements of the hands of a clock or the swings of a pendulum. Very often these movements are only imagined, and the judgment tends to pass into a comparison of durations, one imagined and the other experienced, as when we say " I feel as if I have been out an hour ".

Although the fully formed judgment of duration is one of the latest developments of the sense of time, the rudiments of it go back to very early stages. In certain sea animals which do not seem to have well-marked physiological rhythms, we find variations of behaviour depending on the tides, and these variations continue to occur regularly after the animal is removed to an aquarium.[1] In most animals there is a regular scheme given by heart beats and breathing, and as the speed of these processes is constant, within fairly narrow limits, for each individual or species, the basis of an appreciation of duration is given from birth and low down in the scale of life.

A more conscious experience of rhythm, and consequently of duration, also develops early. Little children can keep time to a march or dance tune, and such dancing to music involves an appreciation of the rhythmic time because we need to *anticipate* the beats. When we fail to anticipate, we cannot " keep time ".

It seems probable that modern civilized man has lost some of the savage capacity for comprehending complicated rhythms. A seven-beat bar is not used in modern music, but appears to occur in some primitive music,[2] and in poetry the tendency of modern verse is on the whole to shorten and simplify the line and stanza. Many of the most exquisite of modern lyrics are of an extreme simplicity and brevity.

The primitive duration experience may in certain cases achieve what appears to be extraordinary exactitude, though we are often unable to decide whether it is really an apprecia-

---

[1] Washburn, *Animal Mind*, 2nd edn., p. 207.
[2] C. S. Myers, *Rhythm in Primitive Music*, B.J. Psy., 1905, p. 397.

tion of duration which is involved or something else. Romanes [1] tells a story of geese who always came into the market on a certain day in the week to pick up scattered grain. One week the market was not held, but the geese came as usual on the regular day. Had the geese judged the lapse of a week, or was Thursday distinguished for them by some special mark ? William James records the case of an idiot girl who always demanded her meals at exactly the same time every day. Her knowledge did not extend to reading the clock, so we are left to wonder if she relied on unwitting estimates of the duration since her last meal, or on other cues afforded by her daily life.[2] The same type of problem arises in connexion with time estimates in sleep, but they will be discussed later.

If then there is an appreciation given by nature of an irreducible minimum of time (the experience that men call the " present " or the " now ") its development up to an appreciation of longer periods depends on memory as a means, the efficient cause, and has the achievement of a purpose as its final cause. Very much the same relation will be found to obtain in the case of the other factors.

We have said that one of the elements which give rise to the idea of pastness is the feeling of familiarity which arises from a memory or a mere recognition of the object. But, as has often been pointed out, this feeling of familiarity is a *present* experience, and therefore logically should not arouse a concept of the past. On the other hand, a present impression (or memory) of something which is past is different from a present impression of something which is

---

[1] *Animal Intelligence*, p. 314.
[2] *Principles of Psychology*, p. 623.

present, or from something which is present but familiar from the past. The distinction between the past and present is that between an image and a perception ; that between the familiar and the unfamiliar, seems to be due to the fact that our reaction to the familiar object is ready, and can proceed without trouble, while we need an effort of thought before to react to the other. If this sense of familiarity is accompanied by an image of the previous occasion on which the object was encountered, we have a complete memory. Among men this feeling of familiarity is generally taken as proof of a previous acquaintance with the object, and referred to some occasion in the past. This is perhaps best observed in those cases of false recollection when we feel convinced that we have experienced all this before and yet can find no warrant for the conviction.

It seems probable, then, that this feeling of familiarity, sometimes strengthened by a memory image, was early used as an indication of past time ; but in itself memory would not have given the past its peculiar qualities. An event which is past may affect our present behavour and thus enter into intimate relation with our purposes, but on the whole, in a primitive state, the past is distinguished from the present by its comparative lack of interest. A dog does not feel the same interest in its last meal as it does in its present one, and " Les nièges d'antan " may be mourned, but do not stir the poet in the same vivid manner as the beauties of his own day.

This being so, it is only natural that the knowledge of, and interest in, the past should increase as our present actions depend more and more on past knowledge and experience. A simple animal capable only of few and stereotyped movements need not refer to the past. A vague feeling of familiarity showing itself in desire for, or aversion from, an object is all that it needs. Memory need not retain the past as an image, and if it were retained, purpose has no use for the knowledge. On the other hand, in man the past is of vital importance for present action. Blot it out for an individual or society, and that individual or society is lost.[1] In intervening stages the past plays a part of ever increasing importance. The higher the animal the more it learns, and therefore the more its activity is guided by the memory of past experience. The needs of exact action force the animal to supplement the vague sense of familiarity by a definite memory image of the past event, and these images, easily distinguished from the present of sense by their character of images, form that body of experience which we call the past.

There is no reason to imagine that at an early stage this past has any definite order within itself. It is not the present because it is an image and the present is perception, nor has it the vivid interest of the present ; it is a general storehouse of images and tendencies to feeling and action, and, just as in a reservoir the water is mingled with little reference to its date of entry, so in this unarranged past the various events need not be grouped in reference to the order in which they entered experience. The two views of the nature of the past can be symbolized in somewhat this manner. A, B, C, D are past events. E is the present

---

[1] Cf. Graham Wallas, *Our Social Heritage.*

moment. If time is arranged as a line these five events lie
thus :—

$$A \to B \to C \to D \to E$$

But there is no need for this arrangement to be linear.
The events can lie thus :—

A
B
C   → E
D

the first four all possess equally the quality of pastness in
regard to E, but are not arranged in degrees of pastness
in reference to each other.

If we may imagine a sea anemone saying in W. James'
words, " Hullo, here's old thingumbob again," we have the
first rudiments of the experience which leads to the concept
of the past. If next minute the same anemone were to
recognize a different, but equally familiar food particle,
thingumgig, there would be the same experience of pastness,
but it would be quite unnecessary for the anemone to decide
in what order thingumbob and thingumgig had previously
entered his experience. Indeed, in adult life, as we shall
see later, the time order presents great difficulties, and a large
part of our own past is not susceptible of arrangement on
a strict time line. We may be able to accomplish such an
arrangement with great difficulty and the aid of dates, but
normally we just dip into our past as into a lucky bag, and
pull out the memory of an event without in the least concerning ourselves about its exact temporal associations.
However, when we wish to think clearly about the past
we import into it the concept of cause and effect, and this

addition necessitates, theoretically at least, an exact and unchanging order of events.

The development of the concept of the future depends mainly on purpose, though memory has some influence on it. It is possible that the concept of the past came into existence before that of the future. A future is only relevant in its earliest stages to some purpose whose end is foreseen but not achieved. For a cat the enjoyment of the saucer of milk which is being slowly lowered from the table is future in a way that its next meal can hardly be to a rudimentary animal. Merely to be hungry does not give us the future, it is a state of the present, but to be hungry and go out to hunt, to sight the quarry, and to chase it—these are acts which make the future for us. In its essence then the future is an unfulfilled purpose which is conscious of its aim.

The definiteness of this aim in part depends on memory. Our anticipations are, in the main, composed of elements provided by memory, since past experience will lend precision to our aim, even though the existence of an aim is not due solely to past experience.

Man's greater powers of imaging or expressing in words the aim of action, or the results of present events, has led to a correspondingly more elaborate organization of the future. It was enough for an animal that the future should be, like the past, without internal organization and arrangement ; man requires for his more complicated purposes that the future shall stretch out in a series in which cause and effect can operate. A cat, doubtless, on setting out at night means to meet other cats, and perhaps howl to the moon ; a man in the same way may go to the club with the intention of seeing his friends ; so far the future is in both cases comparatively formless. It is quite different with calculations of a journey. " I shall catch the 12 o'clock train. That gets to town at 1.10. I have an interview at 2. Therefore I have 20 minutes for lunch at Paddington." Such a plan as this differs widely from the simple intention to go to the club, and the nature of the future demanded by the two plans differs also. There is no reason to imagine that animals have gone beyond their needs in inventing a definite ordered future.

We thus get an organization of the past and future which is in origin strictly utilitarian. The past is the storehouse of knowledge which we use in the present, the future is the accomplishment of our purposes with the different steps leading up to them.

Purpose has appeared as of equal importance with memory in the development of the concepts of duration and of the past and the future ; it is of supreme importance in the unification of time experience and its relation to a single personality. An inactive being would be under little necessity to unify its experience. The sensations of touch and sight might each form a series and these series need not be integrated ; but for an active being, such integration is essential. In our own experience something of the same sort can be observed. It is possible to carry on a train of thought and be conscious of various external physical events without ever fitting the two sets of experiences into a single time scheme. In retrospect they do not form one interpenetrating unity. On the other hand, if we are engaged in some active pursuit we need to integrate the impressions of sight, sound, or touch and direct all our efforts to the one end. In a similar way if experience was originally referred to separate series or " times ", more highly co-ordinated activity must have resulted in its unification ; since it is impossible to pursue an aim which involves nicely adjusted physical action, unless the impressions received from the various senses are related to and form part of a single series of experiences. When this unification had once been accomplished for the individual, the process of generalizing to a unitary world time was comparatively simple. Such a generalization seems, however, to be made anew by each individual, since in the experiments given later we found children who had not yet made it.

In the development of the time concept, therefore, we can roughly distinguish three stages :—(a) a very simple animal whose time perceptions are limited to an experience of duration and to vague feelings of familiarity and appetition ; (b) a complex animal, such as a cat or a dog, which possesses a knowledge of certain marks of time, e.g. meal times or hunting times, has a wider memory of the past, a more definite anticipation of the future, and a unified experience ; and (c) the educated adult, with a social and universal time.

CHAPTER III

SOCIAL ORGANIZATION OF TIME

TIME experience, such as we have described in the last chapter as belonging to the higher animals, is adequate for a being which is going to act in comparative isolation and whose movements are not planned for long periods ahead. Under the conditions of a social life which demands elaborate co-operation, exact methods of time designation are necessary, and, apart from our relations to other men, many of our activities require to be planned long periods in advance.

Thus we get the need for an organized social time reckoning, but this can only be achieved in a certain state of knowledge and by means of certain mechanical devices. It is necessary, therefore, to consider not only the development of time conceptions, but also the history of calendars and clocks. The two topics are closely connected ; since the conscious need called the mechanical devices into existence and these devices reacted on the concepts, enriching them and rendering them more precise.

The aspects of the time of experience which are especially important in society are simultaneity and duration. It is possible to disregard questions concerning the order of events or even of rate of movement, but it is hard to imagine a social organization which does not need to standardize, to some extent, the notions of " when " and " how long ".

Of these two, simultaneity, or synchronization, is much the easier to organize. It is enough to say " we will meet when the sun is a hand's breadth above the horizon ", or " sow your corn when the cranes are heard ". In consequence, the early calendars are based on this principle and the parts of the day are reckoned in a similar manner.

The ordinary individual estimate of duration—as I hope to show below—is subject to the greatest irregularities and is, in almost all cases, unsuitable for use where concerted action is necessary. To organize it we need (a) some external process which appears to proceed with regularity, and (b) some unit into which to divide this process. Neither of these things is particularly easy to achieve, and nature almost appears to have led man designedly astray, since the most obvious means of reckoning—the moon—is in practice unsuitable.

The most primitive forms of time reckoning that we know are essentially unlike those we employ to-day. Our time reckoning is continuous, and presupposes numbered units. We can say " we will meet on 2nd June, 1924 ", or that we will meet in 10 minutes, 6 hours, 3 weeks, 2 months, or 4 years. The older time reckoning frequently does not possess these units ; it does not number those which it does possess. The different possible units are not arranged in relation to each other and, finally, it is unlikely to express itself in duration *periods* but rather to designate a *point* of time.

These points can be clearly illustrated in relation to many periods which seem simple and obvious to us. In the first place, days are more often counted in " nights " than by " suns " or any other designation from the daylight.

This method is "the rule among the primitive Indo-European peoples, the Polynesians, and the inhabitants of North America ".[1] The reason for thus counting the nights is interesting. Among primitive people the tendency in counting time is to count the recurrence of some fixed point rather than a whole duration, apparently because the events which appear to us to be a unity had not been so synthesized. Therefore, in counting days it was not the light time, with its varying occupations, which was considered, but the comparatively durationless night when men lay sound asleep. However, the fact that days were counted in nights did not necessarily mean that this day and night formed a single whole of which one special part was singled out for notice. On the contrary the " day " of 24 hours is a late conception. There are very few words in existence to describe this unit. English does not possess one ; there is a late Greek word νυχθήμερος, a rather artificial German compound " volltag " ; only Swedish apparently having a word " dygn " which has the exact meaning.

Within the day itself the same phenomenon occurs. The day is divided by a series of fixed points, but does not form a series of units of duration. Many tribes have developed a rich terminology to denote the different parts of the day. The names may refer to the sun, as do the Hawaiian terms describing the hours about dawn :—" There comes a glimmer of colour on the mountains," " The curtains of night are parted," " The mountains light up," " Day

---

[1] Martin P. Nilsson, *Primitive Time Reckoning*, p. 15. This valuable book has been extensively used in the following pages, even where an express quotation is not given.

breaks," " The east blooms with yellow," " It is broad
daylight." [1] On the other hand they may be taken from
the occupations or events of daily life. The following list
from Madagascar shows the various kinds of signs in use there.
5.30 p.m. Cattle come home. 5.45 Sunset flush. 6 Sunset.
6.15 The fowls come in. 6.20 Dusk, twilight. 6.45 Edge of
rice-cooking pan obscure. 7 People begin to cook rice.
8 People eat rice. 8.30 Finished eating. 9 People go to
sleep. 9.30 Everyone in bed. 10 Gunfire. 12 Midnight.[2]

In this we have something quite different from our counting of hours. In the first place, as can be seen even from this
selection, the designations cluster more thickly at some
times than at others. At dawn the changes in the light
follow each other rapidly and the beautiful Hawaiian terms
must all refer to a period of about $1\frac{1}{2}$ to 2 hours.

Again, in the list from Madagascar some of the intervals
named are only of 15 minutes, others last 2 hours ; the
period from 5.30 p.m. to 7 p.m. receiving the greatest
number of names. This is the period of sunset when the
sky changes rapidly and animals come home for the night.
The period of sleep is scantily supplied with time designations, and, to a less extent, so is the middle of the day.
It is clear then that these times could not be added to each
other to give longer periods in the way that our hours can.

Furthermore, in many cases, the time indication does not
refer to the duration of the period at all, but to a point
occurring within it. Some of the designations, e.g. the cattle
come home, occupy approximately the whole time till the

[1] D. Mals, *Hawaiian Antiquities*, p. 33.
[2] J. Sibree, *Madagascar before the Conquest*, p. 69.

next designation. Others, as "gunfire", only give a name to a much longer period, which is not otherwise distinguished. This is, of course, different both from our system of frequent and equidistant points of time which are assumed to touch, e.g. 5.10, 5.11, etc., and our reckoning by durations, e.g. half an hour.

Among tribes where so elaborate a nomenclature has not been developed, time indications take an even simpler form, and are given directly by the sun. A native will point to a spot in the heavens and say, we will come when the sun stands there, or that such and such a thing happened when the sun was there. Sometimes a similar method is used, only the judgment is made from the length of shadows. This was often done in Athens, and we can see from Chaucer how long this method lasted and how sophisticated it might become.

> Our Hoste sey wel that the brighte sonne
> Th'ark of his artificial day had ronne
> The fourthe part, and half an houre, and more ;
> And though he was not depe expert in lore,
> He wiste it was the eightetethe day
> Of April, which is messager to May ;
> And sey wel that the shadwe of every tree
> Was as in lengthe the same quantitee
> That was the body erect that caused it.
> And therefore by the shadwe he took his wit
> That Phœbus, which that shoon so clere and bright,
> Degrees was fyve and fourty clombe on highte ;
> And for that day, as in that latitude,
> It was ten of the clokke he gan conclude.

(Chaucer, *Canterbury Tales : Man of Lawe's Prologue.*)

Exactly the same principle of reckoning is used in relation to the year. Just as days are counted in " sleeps " so are years still counted—especially in poetic language—in " winters " or " summers " ; and there are indications that in Europe at one period the unity of the whole year had not been sufficiently well recognized to have a special name. In old German the whole year is often denoted by such expressions as " in bareness and in leaf ", or " in straw and in grass ".[1] In some cases, to be discussed later, a synthesis of the year has never been made.

Within the year, time is indicated at first by a number of seasonal points or short seasons. These points are chosen generally in reference to the life of the people, and may be more or less frequent according to the nature of the events. The Bontoc Igorot, a rice-cultivating people, in some villages reckon eight seasons. They are as follows :—

(1) i-na-na. " No more work in rice sementeras." It lasts about three months.

(2) la-tub. " First harvest." Four weeks.

(3) cho-ok. " Most of rice is harvested." Four weeks.

(4) li-pas. " No more palay-harvest." Ten to fifteen days.

(5) ba-li-ling. " General planting of camotes." Six weeks.

(6) sa-gan-ma. " The seed beds for rice put into condition." Two months.

(7) pa-chong. " Seed-sowing." Though the actual sowing only takes a few days, the period lasts five or six weeks.

(8) sa-ma. " Seedlings planted out." Seven weeks.

[1] Nilsson, op. cit., p. 75.

In this list, which is advanced in character, we get the variations in length of period and the naming of some periods from occupations which do not fill them which occur also in the other lists. The period of seed-sowing in particular extends far beyond the time of the actual work, which is rather an indication of its beginning. In our own case to-day we still use these indications and have the general feeling that spring really begins with the cuckoo or the return of the swallow, that winter is breaking when the catkins come out, that the spider's webs, characteristic of November, mean that autumn is well here, and that the song of the robin heralds winter.

All these time designations are concrete, and there appears to be a great unwillingness to substitute numbers for the descriptive names. This is in part due to a very limited ability to count. Many primitive peoples seem only to count up to small numbers and even when they can count further to avoid doing so as far as possible. There are many methods employed to avoid counting. Among the Negritos of Zambales, the Solomon Islanders, and others, when a feast is arranged for a certain day, the invited guests are given knotted cords, and untie or cut off one knot as each day passes till they come to the proper day for assembling.[1] A similar method is often in use for reckoning months. Other nations use notches in sticks or lay aside a grain of maize, or the stone of a fruit as each day or year passes. When years are counted they are frequently not counted far. The tribes round the southern end of Lake Nyassa reckon in rains up to three or four years ago, everything beyond

[1] Nilsson, op. cit., p. 321.

that is *kale*, " some time ago." [1]   As a result, of course,
few savages count their age.   They may know the year
of their birth, marked by some outstanding event, or their
age relative to some other person, but do not know how many
years they have lived.

The unwillingness or inability to count is all the more
striking among tribes who have developed elaborate names
for the different days of such a period as the moon month.
In Micro- and Polynesia many tribes have names for most
of the days of the moon month, or for small groups of two
or three days throughout the month, but the days are not
numbered.

Even when the days do begin to be numbered, the month
is generally divided into sections so as to decrease the
magnitude of the numbers used.   This stage is illustrated
by the Greek division of the month into ἱστάμενος and
φθίνων and the Roman counting of so many days before the
Nones, Ides (the full moon), and Kalends (the new moon).

If counting was adopted with such reluctance and so
late, it explains why primitive peoples find it so hard to
discard the concrete point reckoning of time and to adopt
continuous units.   This is best illustrated by the stages in
the evolution of the year.   Among a people which recognizes the different seasons, it would seem a natural step to
combine the whole cycle of these seasons, and start a new
year when a particular season came round ; but in many
cases this has not been done.   In the Bismarck Archipelago
there are monsoon years of five months, the two intervening
periods of the variable winds and calms (each lasting one

[1] Ibid., p. 97.

month) are not counted.[1] In Brazil certain of the peoples count only 6 months to the year, though one season is wet and the other dry. In North Asia six-month periods are reckoned as separate " years ", being called winter years and summer years.

Sometimes the arrangement is even more curious. The years, instead of being simply bisected solar years, contain a number of months which does not divide into the solar year, e.g. they may consist of 9, 10, or 11 months. This may occur, as in the Marquesas, even when the people are able to recognize the sidereal year by the rising of the Pleiades. These short years seem to be caused by an exclusive attention to the phenomena of agriculture. They are vegetation years, and are reckoned from sowing to harvest ; the period in which no agricultural work is done is simply passed over. As a result, of course, the years are not continuous, and the metaphysical difficulties of where one year ends and the other begins need not trouble anyone.[2]

A continuous form of time reckoning is first clearly suggested by the moon, though in the most primitive cases the days of invisibility are neglected, thus rendering the months discontinuous after the manner of vegetation years. The moon month, however, is a fairly short period, and the continuity of one month with another is soon recognized. This organization of the moon month as a unit, while the year was still unsettled, led to one of the greatest difficulties in the history of the calendar. If there were exactly 12 or

[1] G. Brown, *Melanesians and Polynesians*, p. 331.
[2] Rose Macaulay, *Told by an Idiot*, p. 170. " The funny thing was that you could not, however hard, . . ." etc.

13 moon months in the year all would have been well, but there are not, and a date in a year which counts only 12 months will go the whole round of the seasons in 33 years. In consequence, at a stage where the concrete phenomena of nature are of supreme importance in relation to time reckoning, some adjustment has to be made. This is exceedingly difficult, since it means abandoning either the moon or the vegetation seasons. But when, as frequently happens, the months are named after phases of animal or vegetable life, it has to be done, since it is impossible for the literal-minded savage to call a month " the moon of strawberries " at a time when the strawberries have not even flowered.

As a consequence, the earliest form of intercalation arises. When, in the opinion of the tribe in council, the strawberries are not sufficiently advanced to justify the present month being named after them, this month is " forgotten " and the following month receives the name which corresponds with the actual vegetation. This form of intercalation was systematized among the Jews, and was necessary because at the Passover the first fruits of corn were offered. The court of justice visited the fields, and if the corn and fruit did not appear sufficiently advanced, thirty days were by decree inserted in the year.

Such intercalation may degenerate into a political weapon, as it did among the Romans, and the only way to escape from it is to dissociate the year from the moon. The length of the year is then generally determined by the rising of some constellation, usually the Pleiades, or more rarely by the equinoxes or solstices. Even when dissociated from the moon, the months still tend to be connected with concrete natural phenomena. An interesting proof of this is afforded by the way in which the Julian months have been renamed in many popular calendars in Europe (e.g. Lithuanian, Lettish, Czech, Croat, etc.) to suit national seasons. In England children still love the old rhymes which connect the months with changes in weather or animals.

One nation seems to have achieved the task of dissociating its calendar completely from nature. The Egyptians had a year of 12 months of 30 days each and 5 extra days. They consequently disregarded the moon in their calculations. They had also three seasons : " inundation," " seed time," and " harvest ". Owing to the long time for which their calendar ran, and the neglect of the fraction of the day in the year, the calendar got out of place in relation to the Nile. It therefore happened that the season of " inundation " by the calendar might coincide with the actual harvest. This, however, does not appear to have been considered serious, and the morning rising of Sirius, which was theoretically the beginning of the year, was celebrated as a movable feast in relation to the calendar, which was thus free both from the moon and vegetation seasons.

Supposing that a people have arrived at the length of a year, there is a further point to be settled—when shall the year begin ? The most obvious method, especially with an agricultural people, is to start the year with the beginning or end of the period of cultivation. On the whole, the end of the cultivation period is most often chosen as the time of the new year, because the new food supplies are then at hand, and the year can open in abundance with offerings.

This is no more a fixed date than is our own period of harvest thanksgiving, but in a rude calendar it is quite satisfactory. The seasons of the Bontoc Igorot given above, illustrate the beginning of the year with a period of rest and plenty. It may happen that a people has more than one important crop, and in that case we find "new years" corresponding to the harvest homes of the different food stuffs.

A far more accurate way of beginning the year is by observations of the sun or stars.   The rising of the Pleiades, and generally the evening rising, is one of the most favoured methods of determination, and the number of legends connected with them testify to the popularity of these stars. The Eskimos start their year from the winter solstice, and other peoples have chosen different periods.   In general, we can say that there is no natural beginning to the year, but it is chosen at such time as is convenient to each people ; and in rare cases, the calendar year may be even dissociated entirely from the natural year and celebrate its " new year " at various points in the vegetation cycle.[1]

The last stage in the organization of the calendar is the arrangement of the years in a numbered series.   This does not, of course, take place as long as there is an aversion to using numbers, especially large ones.   In place of numbers, the years are distinguished by striking events which have occurred in them.   These lists of events may be highly developed and extend for many years.   The Herrero had a calendar of this kind reaching from 1820 till about 1900, when the growing influence of Europeans destroyed this method of reckoning.   In some tribes the history of the

[1] We to-day have at least 4 "years" starting at different times : the scholastic, the financial, the calendar, and the ecclesiastical.

people is recorded by notches on a stick or by pictures, and the calendar-man can interpret the notches or pictures, giving the history of the people. A reckoning of this sort has in one case been systematized into a sort of cycle. The Batak of Sumatra believe that there is a small-pox epidemic at intervals of from nine to twelve years. If a man has been alive for two such epidemics, he is assumed to be about 20 years old.[1] This form of reckoning reaches its most civilized form in states which have yearly changing magistrates. The consuls at Rome and the archons at Athens gave their names to the years, and enabled a complete and homogeneous list of years to be drawn up. The disadvantages of this method are obvious. It requires a very good memory to keep in mind the complete list, and failing that, the mere dating by consuls does not give the power to arrange the years in order. The Romans therefore supplemented their dating by consuls by giving the years A.U.C., and the Greeks by their reckoning in Olympiads.

A halfway stage between the pure designation of the year by its events and the numbered series is reached when the years of a reign are counted ; but this method is not employed immediately there is a stable monarchy. The earliest method is to name the year of the king's accession after him, " The year of King So-and-So," and then name the other years of his reign after important events as before. This was apparently the method employed in Babylonia in the days of the Sumerian Kingdom of Ur, and under the first dynasty in Babylon.[2]

In Egypt, after this stage, the simple counting of the

---

[1] Hose and McDougall, *Pagan Tribes of Borneo*, ii, 214.
[2] L. W. King, *History of Babylon*, p. 215.

years of the King's reign appears, and from the end of the
old Kingdom completely supplants the other method ;
but frequently these years are not calendar years, but run
from the date of the King's accession. At certain periods,
however, these years were counted from New Year's Day,
and so coincided with the calendar year. The invention of
the era is thus the last step, and when this has been made,
and its general convenience recognized, the development of
the calendar on this side is complete.

So far we have been working up from the day, and only
treated the subdivisions of the day incidentally as
illustrations of the principle of discontinuous reckoning ;
but as soon as time was conceived as something continuous
the subdivision of the day was undertaken. In this men were
as dependent on measuring devices as they had been
dependent on astronomy in finding the correct length of the
year. The need to determine the year came early, since
agriculture and sailing were both interested in it ; the
subdivisions of the day were not felt to be necessary for a
long time, and the need for an exact chronometer was not
acknowledged till the days of Dr. Johnson, when Parliament
offered a prize for one to assist in navigation.

The day, like the year, presents serious difficulties to the
systematizer. The most obvious and the earliest method
was to take the period of daylight and subdivide that into
a certain number of " hours ". But if the number of subdivisions was kept at 12, the hours would vary in length,
summer and winter. This was the condition of things in
Greece, and it was so well recognized that special devices
were invented for making the water-clock indicate these

hours of varying length. The night, on the other hand, was, at this period, not divided into hours, but simply into four " watches ".

The natural line of advance was to reckon from sunrise to sunrise, and divide the whole period into 24 hours, but even so, for exact calculation there are difficulties, due to the obliquity of the ecliptic, the eccentricity of the earth's orbit, and the differences between the lengths of the solar and stellar day. The result is that, for astronomy, there are four days. There are two sidereal days, reckoned by the transits of the first point of Aries and by the transits of any other fixed star. These days are very nearly the same, being only about $\frac{1}{100}$ sec. different. The solar day is roughly 4 minutes longer than the stellar day, and it can be calculated either on the movements of the sun, as seen at any point, or on the movements of an imaginary body, the " mean sun ", which are averaged over a " tropical year ". The relation between the true and mean noon at any point is constantly changing, the one first preceding and then succeeding the other, and, on occasion, the difference may be considerable. If, therefore, the day is to be accurately divided, considerable astronomical knowledge and apparatus are necessary. In spite of this, a fairly good approximation to equal hours was popularized in the thirteenth and fourteenth centuries by the use of striking clocks. The early clocks which we possess are provided with striking gear, and their general use in churches must have accustomed people to a regular continuous time reckoning.

The farther history of time measurement is the gradual stabilization of the periods and their subdivision. The factor which most strongly influenced the former was navigation, which demanded a reliable chronometer for the calculation of longitude, while the latter was the concern of science, which was continually demanding the means for measuring more and more minute subdivisions of time. As the power to measure these subdivisions has increased, so has our sense of time become more precise. It is no harder for a scientist to-day to think in $\frac{1}{1000}$ of a second than it must have been for the mediæval ploughman to think in hours. It is perhaps easier, for the idea of exact time measurement has grown so familiar to us, so much an integral part of our daily lives, that a watch which loses two minutes a day fills us with disgust, and it is only in some dream or happy holiday island that we get rid of the perpetual lurking thought of the clock.

CHAPTER IV

INDIVIDUAL ORGANIZATION OF TIME

THE evolution of a scheme of conventional time such as I have sketched in the last chapter was a work of ages. The ordinary inhabitant of a civilized country learns to use this scheme during childhood, and, by the time he reaches maturity, should be master of the whole complicated arrangement of hours, days, and years.

Little children are notoriously ignorant and incapable where time is concerned, and Binet included questions on time in his Intelligence Tests. In his 1906 scale he ascribed to children of 6 years the knowledge whether it is morning or afternoon, and to those of 9 years the knowledge of the day of the week, the month, the day of the month, and the year. At 10 he supposed children to be able to repeat the names of the months correctly.[1] Burt in his study of reasoning in children,[2] comments on the great difficulty they seem to find in making " time syntheses ".

Most of the studies of children's knowledge of time are concerned with little children, and are based on a consideration of their vocabularies ; the supposition being that from children's use of words their concepts can be deduced.

The most complete study of a child's use of time words is that of Decroly and Degan,[3] but other writers on childhood,

---

[1] Binet, *Development of Intelligence in Children*, Engl. Transl. (1916), pp. 206–17.

[2] *Jl. of Exp. Ped. Dec.*, 1919.

[3] Decroly et Degan, *Archives de Psychol.*, 1913.

especially Stern [1] and Preyer,[2] have given information
about it.

The earliest words or indications of time knowledge
refer, naturally, to the present, and are concerned with
simultaneities, e.g. S. (the child observed by Decroly and
Degan) knew at 1 year 4 months when the entrance of a
person foretold a bath, which she loved, or time to lie down,
which she disliked. She rapidly learnt when she might
expect to be given a sweet (2.2) ; the order of events in the
day, and the bells which marked them (2.3 ; 2.11) ; and at
3 years expressed surprise if the customary order was
changed. With Stern's child, Hilda, the present is the first
division of time to be given a name.

The past appears to be next distinguished. By 1.10 and
2 years S. used " Voilà " or " Pati " to show that she had
finished something, and by 2.1 she used the past participle
in reference to the past, and at the same age seemed to have
an idea of an immediate past. By 2.6 her memory for past
events extended to 15 days.

According to Stern, the infinitive is used at first to cover
past, present, and future ; Decroly does not note its use
for the future till the age of 2.5, and at the same time the
idea of a future act arises, but only when it is suggested by
the sight of some object connected with it, e.g. trying on
new clothes recalls to S., when once it has been suggested,
the pleasures of a journey in the train and a visit. The
other time concepts develop later, particular difficulty being
felt over the relativity of such terms as " to-morrow " and

[1] Stern, *Die Kindersprache*, 1907.
[2] Preyer, *Die Seele des Kindes*, 1905.

" to-day ". When children reach school age and have learnt to speak readily and write their own language it is possible to investigate more closely the various ideas that they have formed of time, and the extent to which they have mastered the use of the various time symbols and designations common to their country. If it can be shown that the stages in which conventional time designations are learnt correspond roughly to the stages in which they were invented, it can be assumed that the use of time marks corresponds to some mental power which gradually develops in the individual and the race, and follows approximately the same course in both.

The following experiments were undertaken primarily with an educational aim, and this in part accounts for their form, but as they illustrate the development of the individual knowledge of time they are inserted here.[1] The connexion of the findings of the experiment with the stages of primitive time organization will be pointed out at the end. The experiments were directed to investigating :—

(i) The child's understanding of ordinary time-words and symbols such as are used in everyday life.

(ii) His power to form the conception of a universal time scheme extending into the past and future, and his ability to use the dates which symbolize this scheme.

(iii) His knowledge of the characteristics of definite epochs in the time scheme, and his ability to place these epochs roughly in their correct order.

(iv) The matter and methods used by the child in thinking about historical data.

---

[1] I must thank Miss Oakden for allowing me to reproduce this paper, of which she is part author. It appeared in the *B. J. of Psy.*

(v) The importance attached by children to time in comparison with other elements in their experience.

The tests used were :—

A. A list of questions intended to illustrate (i) and (ii) above.

B. Lists of historical characters with dates, dealing with (ii) above.

C. An absurdity test, two completion tests, and the arrangement of people in order, in their centuries and in epochs. The last of these tests had two forms : (a) the names of people were given ; (b) pictures were shown. All these were used to illustrate (iii) and (iv) above.

D. A memory test and the composition of a letter, dealing with (v) above.

The " questions " test

This test was always given individually and orally when given to the younger children. To one set of older children, ages 8–10, it was given in class as a group test, and the answers were written.

The following is a list of the questions asked :—

1. What is your age ?
2. What is the date of your birthday, (a) month, (b) day of month ?
3. Is it morning or afternoon ? Why ?
4. What day of the week is it ?
5. How long would it take you to walk round this room ?
6. What season is it ? Why ?
7. What month is it ?
8. What day of the month is it ?
9. What year is it ?
10. In what year were you born ?
11. What day is it at [e.g. Newmarket] now ?
12. What time is it now ?
13. What time is it for your mother at home ?

14. Robin Hood lived in 1187. (a) Would your mother be alive then ? (b) Would your grandmother ?
15. Would Christ be alive then ?
16. How long is it since the [e.g. Easter] holidays ?
17. At what time does School begin ?
18. At what time does School end ?
19. Will you come to School on Saturday ?
20. How long will it be till holidays begin again ?
21. (a) When you are [e.g. 10], will you be older or younger ? (b) Will your mother be older, younger, or the same ?
22. How long have you been talking to me ?

In answer to Q. 5 two estimates were required, the second (called 5b) after the child had actually walked round the room. Q. 13 was always introduced by : " Has your mother a clock at home ? " and " Is it right ? " It was actually asked in the form : " What time would she see if she looked at it now ? " Q. 14 was asked thus : " Have you heard of Robin Hood ? " If the answer was " No ", the experimenter said : " He was a robber and lived in the forests. He lived in the year 1187. Was your mother alive then ? "

In marking, four symbols were used : R = right ; W = wrong ; — = no answer ; ! = an absurd answer. The marking of most of the questions presented no difficulty, but a few questions need special mention.

Qs. 8 and 9 had to be quite right. The children were told the date in school.

Q. 12. Five or ten minutes' latitude was allowed.

Qs. 16 and 20. Estimates with more than a week's error were counted as wrong.

Q. 22. An answer of five or ten minutes counted right (the tests actually took about 7 minutes) ; a greater or less time, e.g. 2 or 15 minutes, was counted wrong.

Such answers as the following were counted as " absurd ".

Q. 5. Five minutes or over.

Q. 6. Any answer that was quite wrong, e.g. " Nearly July, because the apples are on the trees ". It was March. Any answer that was reasonable, e.g. " Summer, because it is so hot " (the day being a particularly hot one in March), was counted as right.

Qs. 7 and 9. Any answer apparently senseless, e.g. 3.

Q. 12. A time more than two hours out, or some repeated phrase that seemed to mean nothing.

Qs. 16 and 20. All periods much too long or too short, e.g. 5 days instead of about 2 months, or 6 or 12 months instead of 2 months.

Qs. 17 and 18. Any time more than one hour out.

Q. 22. Any time more than half-an-hour out.

The table on p. 49 shows the percentage of children answering each question rightly (R), absurdly (!), and failing to answer (—), at each age. The percentage of children answering wrongly (W) is not shown, but can readily be calculated. The questions are arranged in order of increasing difficulty.

In estimating the ages at which the various questions can be answered, it is perhaps best to consider the columns giving absurdities and failure to answer. The 4-year-old children know very little, and their absurdities are mainly in answers to those questions which involve giving the time of day. At 5 years of age the greater number of absurdities is to be found in the answers to questions on duration ; while from 7 onwards the absurdities have largely disappeared, thus showing, on our system of marking, a certain general

TABLE I

No. and nature of question	4 (14) R	!	–	5 (12) R	!	–	6 (15) R	!	–	7 (13) R	!	–	8 (25) R	!	–	9 (25) R	!	–	10 (6) R	!	–
Age	100			100			100			100			100			100			100		
19. School on Saturday	78	·	7	91			100			100			96			100			100		
3. Morning	67			83			100			100			100			100			100		
22. When 10 you older	50	43		75			80			100			92			100			80		
2. Birthday : month	50		29	50		50	73		20	100		8	92		8	88			100		
4. Day of week	21		50	73		9	87		7	77			96		8	92			100		
14. R. H. : mother	50			66			67		13	84		8	97			92			100		
13. Time for mother	50		29	75			60		7	84			92			92			67		
21. When 10 mother older	14	43	21	42			87		15	82			84			100			100		
18. What time return from school	7	35	43	33	25	16	54			82		31	88		7	100			100		
2. Birthday : day of month	7		86	25		75	27		60	69		16	91			84		8	86		
11. Day in other town	7		21	58			60			54		27	96		7	100			100		
7. Month	14		78	8		66	20	13	33	77		53	64	4	8	84		8	86		
6. Season	7	7	78	50		42	31	8	54	27	9		83		8	100			100		
14. R. H. : grandmother	35			58			40		7	38		8	83		8	96			67		
6. Season. Why	14		78	63		35	30	10	40	9		64	63		12	89			100		
17. Time school begins	7	43	29	16	25	16	46		7	45			74	7	4	82	4		83		
9. Year	·	14	86	8		91	7	13	80	46		46	53		8	96			100		
15. R. H. : Jesus Christ	14		7	33		16	54		7	54		54	84		4	92	4		30		
8. Day of month	·	7	93	·		66	7		73	31		16	28		8	12		8	57		
16. How long since the holidays	14	7	71	8	33	25	27	27	13	31		8	48		4	80	8		23		
22. Time been talking	·	7	78	25	33		20	7	13	46	16	38	34	3	8	36	8		29		14
20. How long till holidays	·	14	64	·		100	31	15	31	·		32	30	6	6	36	8		71		
10. When born	7	7	93	·	16	33	33	7	20	18		46	47	6	13	56	12	13	43		
12. Time now	·	35	64	8	33	16	·	27	7	38			38	7	10	12	8	10	14		
5. How long to walk round (a)	·	·	86	·	33	8	7	27	40	·	8	·	22	7	·	8	12	·	14	16	
5. ,, ,, (b)	·	21	64	·	12		7	27		·	8		10	13		4	16		·	14	

E

knowledge of the terms involved. The 10-year-old group
is small and came from a class in which the average age was
9 ; it therefore consisted of children below the average
intelligence of the class. In spite of this, the 10-year-old
group is on the whole better than the 9-year-old group, and
shows a fairly close approximation to the adult knowledge
of time.

There seems to be a slight change in the order of difficulty
of the questions at different ages. This may well be due to
the smallness of the groups investigated. Accidental
factors have undoubtedly affected the position of certain
questions.[1]

To arrange the questions in order of difficulty, and thus
to determine the order of the growth of knowledge, is
difficult. Some facts, however, seem clear. The duration
questions are clearly the hardest, so much so that they are
beyond the power of most adults to answer correctly.
E.g. Q. 5 was only answered correctly by one adult out of
seven tested, and he was an amateur photographer practised
in estimating short periods of time. The difficulty of Qs.
16 and 20 for the children seemed to be partly due to their
inability to perform the necessary calculations, such as
would be made by an adult if he could not tell " off-hand "
the length of time before a certain event. It is noteworthy
that only one of the younger children made use of organized
experience, saying, " I suppose the term will be three months;
it usually is."

[1] Cf. Q. 15 ; the children of the school which wrote the answers to these
questions had clearly been taught that Jesus lives *eternally*, wherefore in
almost all cases they said that He was alive at the same time as Robin
Hood.

Next in degree of difficulty may be put the questions involving the time of day. Q. 12 is probably too hard for most adults ; the man who can tell the time correctly without looking at his watch being generally regarded as something rather out of the common. It is noteworthy that Q. 17 proves to be much harder than Q. 18. It might be thought that this is due to the children tending to confuse the time of leaving home with that of the actual beginning of school, but for the fact that they give a time that is late quite as often as one that is early. Knowledge of other points seems to grow irregularly ; though the tendency is for growth to occur outwards from the more to the less personally interesting, and from frequently recurring cycles to those of longer periodicity.

Both the day of the month and the year involve counting, and this does not become easy and habitual until a child is about 7 or 8 years old.[1] The season seems to children much less a mark of time than a description of concrete material things that enter directly into their experience. Winter really means for them snow, or Spring, flowers. Consequently, a wrong season may be given with the right description ; on a very warm March day Q. 6 may produce many answers such as " Summer, because it is so hot ". This also explains the greater difficulty children find in giving a reason for their thinking it is morning or afternoon. When a reason was given, and not merely the intuitionist's " I just know ", it usually concerned personal activity, often a meal. Such answers as " The sun is setting " occur, but rarely.

[1] Ballard, *Mental Tests*, pp. 55, 62, 71.

Perhaps the most interesting results are those bearing on the universal nature of time. Most children realize quite early that time is the same all over the same town (Q. 13 can be answered by 50 per cent of the 4-year-old children), and also that the sequence of time in the future for others is the same as for themselves (v. Q. 21). But even at 10 years of age the fact that time is (practically) the same in different English towns is not realized in all cases. One 8-year-old who knew that it was Saturday in Cambridge, summed up the matter quite finally, " It would be Sunday in London, 'cos it's a different town, and there are towns where it would be Monday." She was pressed for an example, " It would be Monday in Hunstanton, 'cos that is different again." Of course, children seldom express themselves as definitely as this, but in cases where it has been possible to get the child to give a reason at all for his answer he seems to think as did the child quoted. A difficulty may arise for him from his observation of the fact that different people's timetables vary greatly ; " baby " goes to bed at a time different from " sister " or " mother ". Even when " time " is thought of as being the same within a child's circle of experience, why should it be so in places which are apparently so entirely disconnected from it ?

Binet commented on the fact that children found great difficulty in naming the year, a task which appears easy to adults. This knowledge seems to be acquired suddenly, and in a way rather different from that of the other elements of the date. From 4–6 years of age there is practically no knowledge of the year. At 7 about half know, and from 8–10 nearly all. It was, however, far from certain that, because the children could give the year as part of the date, they had any real understanding of a chronological system. When they were asked to give the year of their birth the highest percentage of successful answers was 56 at age 9 ; but at that age, and still more at 10, the children ought to have been able to make the needed calculation if they had understood the principle on which dates were arranged. The other question, 14, intended to test an appreciation of dates, did not seem to give results at all conclusive. It appeared to be Robin Hood's name, rather than the date, that suggested a period remote from ordinary experience. The description given of him as a robber, and the stories of him in the books where he was often described as living in " the olden times ", probably often determined the right answer when it was given. If the children had made any calculation, even the simplest, there would not have been so much difference between the answers in the cases of their mothers and grandmothers (Q. 14a and b). Apparently, grandmother's experience could be so remote that anything might have happened in those days. One quite clever and well-taught child of 8½, who answered practically all the questions rightly, was quite unable to decide about her grandmother. " You see," she said, " Granny lived to be 80." She never made any attempt to obtain an answer from calculation. Another child, aged 6, placed Robin Hood exactly a generation back. " Mother was a baby in his time, like I am now, and Granny was a young lady, like Mother is." Many other children said that he lived at a time different from Christ, but when asked whether it was before or after, they replied " before ".

The " order of dates " test

The " questions " test showed that children make very little use of dates. This might be due to inability to perform the necessary calculations, or to ignorance of the significance of the dates themselves. We therefore have the following test in various schools, viz. the two lowest forms of a Girls' High School, X, a Boys' Preparatory School, Y, and two Elementary Schools, A and B, the latter in a slum district. We must thank all these schools for their kindness in allowing us to carry out this and other tests.

On the blackboard was written :

Attila lived in Hungary in A.D. 438.

Philip lived in Spain in A.D. 1585 (or *Dante lived in Florence in* A.D. 1312).

Nero lived in Rome in A.D. 50.

This was read out to the children and they were told to write down the names of the people in the order in which they lived, " beginning with the one who lived longest ago— furthest away back in history." The test was performed slowly, and additional explanations were given if they were asked for. When the children had done this a similar test was given containing the names of Plato, Burke, and Swift. In its earliest form the test contained five names ; but as only 20 per cent of the children tested, aged 10, were capable of answering, we thought that the number should be reduced to three. The results given are for the shorter form shown above.

Ability to perform the test varied considerably at the different schools. School Y was slightly superior at all ages,

TABLE II

	Attila series		*Burke* series	
Age	No. of children	% answering correctly	No. of children	% answering correctly
8	45	51	45	69
9	75	61	56	71
10	57	67	40	93
11	52	89	40	93
12	40	85	37	92
13	28	96	25	100

though the children were rather hurried ; B was much the worst.

The highest scores in the second test are mainly due to the fact that school B did not take it ; but as all the schools show a slight improvement in it, a few of the errors in the first test may be due to the unfamiliarity of the task. The majority of the errors, however, show real ignorance. They were mainly inversions ; and when reasons were demanded the most usual reply was, " Philip comes first because his number is bigger." This error was, however, complicated by the fact that some children did not know when the number *was* bigger; e.g. in the problem below, 1898 was often thought to be bigger than 1901. Indeed, some children seemed to judge of the value of a date by its last figure.[1] Other mistakes arose through ignorance of " B.C.", one child thinking that it came after " A.D."; but, on the whole, there were fewer mistakes due to this than might have been expected.[2] The utter confusion of a few of the children can be gathered from the following answers to questions. M. D., aged 10, school A : " Nero lived 50 years ago, Dante

[1] This is partly explained by the fact that this school adopts the modern idea of dealing with *small* numbers in arithmetical calculations. Numbers greater than 1,000 are therefore unfamiliar.
[2] Cf. " pictorial identification " test, later.

1312, therefore Dante lived first." M. E., 9, A : " Look at Dante and Nero, whose date is later ? " " Dante's." " Who lived longest ago then ? " " Dante." P. M., 10, A : " Why do you think Attila lived after Philip ? " " I just guessed, I had nothing to guide me."

The majority of children seemed vague as to the point from which years are enumerated ; and even where " B.C." was understood, did not realize whether this point was in the future or past.

It was suggested by one teacher that the children failed because of the unfamiliar names and the remoteness of the dates. We therefore gave a problem to some of the same children which was free from these objections. It ran :

John was born in 1898, Mary was born in 1901. Who is the older ?

The results of this test were better than those of the other. With the same children they were :

Age	Per cent answering correctly the *Attila-Burke* series	Per cent answering correctly the *John-Mary* problem
8	48	67
9	57	70
10	50	71

If this difference is due to the cause suggested, it would be another example of the difficulty that children find in generalizing their time-knowledge.

The " temporal absurdities " test

The two tests above described show that only from about 9 years of age can the majority of children be assumed to possess a knowledge of the conventional scheme of time-marking used in everyday life and in history. Even at that age it is quite unsafe to assume that much more than a half of the class understands the principle on which chronology is based, or what is intended to be conveyed when the date of some historical character is given.

But dates are merely the scaffolding of history, and an understanding of them is quite distinct from a knowledge of the characteristics of the different periods which they denote. It seems probable that the power to understand this depends partly on age, even apart from the effects of different methods of teaching. We were told by an experienced teacher that she had given up telling stories about the remote historic past to children of 7 because they seemed quite unable to imagine a state of things when there were no trains or when the servant's " night out " did not have to be considered. At 8 she found that they could manage this. Given this power to think of the past as different from the present, there still seem to be at least two stages in the development of historical knowledge. The first may be called the " negative " stage ; at this stage the present is distinguished from the past by the qualities which the latter *lacks* rather than those which it possesses. Each child sums up the *positive* characteristics of the past, as it appears to him, in some short formula such as wearing sandals and skins or worshipping idols. He relegates whatever seems to him to be beyond his own experience, or the possible experience of those with whom he comes into close contact, to the dim regions of " savagery ".

The second stage occurs only when the child begins to distinguish historical periods, and to form a picture of *successive* epochs approximating to that formed by an adult.

The following absurdity test was devised to examine the

child's power of distinguishing a historical epoch from the present ; and also his power of using effectively such knowledge as was investigated by the " questions " and " order of date " tests.

In 55 B.C. Julius Cæsar arrived with his troops at Dover. They had had a stormy crossing, and now, as the sun was sinking, they splashed through the surf to the land. The Britons on the shore were singing at

A

their mid-day meal, and did not notice the noise the Romans made until

B

the enemy forces were only a quarter of a mile away. A day's march brought the Britons to the spot. The next day, Wednesday, the

C

30th February, the Romans caught a British prisoner. He told them the British troops were discontented, as they wished to go home at once

D

to reap their autumn harvest. Cæsar was greatly encouraged and forced a battle the next day. At dawn he offered a sacrifice. Taking

E   F

off his top-hat he stood before the Altar, and prayed " O, Lord Jesus,

G

may this day, Friday, by others regarded as unlucky, prove fortunate to us." The Romans won a great victory, due to their superiority in

H

gun fire. The British chieftain was taken prisoner and shown in Cæsar's

K

triumphal procession three years later, 58 B.C. His grandson is

L

still living in a remote corner of Scotland.

This test was given with the instructions : " Here is a story. In it are many things which are wrong, nonsense, or absurd. You are to underline all the things that you can find wrong or absurd and to write in the margin why you think them so." An example was then given.[1] The actual test was given to school Y (cf. p. 54) throughout,[2] to two

[1] It was taken from the absurdity test given in Ballard, *Mental Tests*, p. 38.
[2] It was impossible to test the top mathematical form at Y. This meant that only two of the top classical form did the tests. As the school is predominantly classical, the cleverer 13-year-olds and some of the best 12-year-olds did not do the tests. The absence of these boys influences the results of the " J.C." test and "completion " test.

forms of school A, ages 8–11, and to forms I, II, and III of
a Bristol Central School, ages 11–14. The results may be
tabulated :

			Percentage of children scoring each point					
Age	8	9	10	11	12	13	14	
No. of								
children	26	51	71	55	65	66	24	Total Average
A	27	47	49	78	86	79	88	454 65
B	8	18	30	60	66	48	75	305 44
C	35	25	8	33	37	29	21	188 27
D	27	33	41	64	66	76	50	357 51
E	50	49	54	73	83	86	83	478 67
F	15	16	25	44	48	39	58	245 35
G	23	35	34	54	48	53	46	293 42
H	31	37	59	80	95	94	100	496 71
K	27	20	20	42	43	38	12	202 29
L	42	47	61	89	89	83	83	494 70
Average	28·5	32·7	38·1	61·7	66·1	62·5	61·6	

If one considers the results obtained by children at
different ages the most noticeable fact is the sharp improvement between the ages of 10 and 11. Both above and below
that age there is but little improvement ; at that point the
score practically doubles. The results of school Y are
markedly superior to those of the other schools, the average
score in this case for all ages being 56 per cent, and in all
the other schools together being 42·1 per cent. In spite of
this, however, the order of difficulty of the points is practically identical. This shows that the test presented the same
characteristic difficulties to each group, although the boys
of school Y were more competent to deal with them.

If we range the points in their order of difficulty, the
easiest first, they run :

H Gun fire.

L Grandson still alive.

E Cæsar's top-hat.

A Sun-set and midday meal.

D Autumn harvest.

B Day's march.

G Friday following Wednesday.

F Christ worshipped in B.C.

K 58 B.C. 3 years after 55 B.C.

C 30th of February.

We can divide these points roughly into three classes. H, I., E emphasize the distinction between the past and the present, and are the easiest. A, D, B come next and have to do with time as measured by reference to natural phenomena or personal activity. The last four points, G, F, K, C, exemplify purely conventional marks of time. If we compare these results with those obtained from the " questions " test (pp. 46–53), the correspondence is, on the whole, remarkably close. In the " questions " test the " day of the month " is one of the hardest—almost the hardest if we exclude the very difficult " duration " questions ; while in the above absurdity test C proves the hardest point. In both tests, points relating to the year and to the connexion of Christ with the beginning of the A.D. period occur next in order of difficulty. Points requiring a knowledge of the different seasons and the power to realize, however vaguely, when a period passes the span of life of a grandfather or grandson, came third in order of difficulty. All this seems to show that there is actually a definite order in which these elements of knowledge are acquired, and that this order can be demonstrated in different types of material.

While this test thus confirms the results of the "questions" test, it also supports the view that the earliest distinction the child makes is between the present and a historical past which is as different as possible from that present. This was shown to some extent by the reasons given by the children for marking the various points in the absurdity test. In addition to those points which the experimenter intended to be observed, many others were marked as absurd that were not meant to appear so, e.g. dating by our calendar. The comments made show a gradual change in type. Those of the younger children almost always run : " They did not have dates." " The Britons had no troops." The past appears to be considered simply as negating existing practices. As the children grow older, a positive standard of judgment appears. " Cæsar had a helmet, and therefore could not wear a top-hat." Or, " They did not know about dates and days till the English came." In one case a boy gave a long, and quite correct, account of the Roman calendar. This change is noteworthy, and seems to occur mainly about 11 years of age.

The " temporal completion " test

To investigate further the positive differentiation of epochs we used at first two " completion " tests. The children were given sentences dealing with the dress and social life of the Romans and of the English in the time of Charles I, and were asked to complete the sentences correctly. The marking was necessarily difficult, but it was all carried out by one person, and every effort was made to keep it uniform. The papers were marked in five grades G (good), F +, F (fair), F - , B (bad). To be B the completion had to bear no reference to the period indicated, e.g. attributing to the reign of Charles I the mud huts and human sacrifices of the ancient Britons. F showed a passable, though generally vague knowledge of the period, G a really definite one.

The following is one of the blanks used. The other was exactly the same, save that it dealt with the Romans.

1. The occupations of the English in the time of Charles I were....
   ....
2. Their food consisted of.......................................
3. They lived in houses made of................................
4. Their chief city was..
5. When they went to war the weapons they used were.........
   ....
6. When they were at peace they wore on their bodies............
7. On their heads they wore ....
8. On their feet they wore.......................................
9. They worshipped...........and to please him they...........
   ....
10. The language they spoke was................................
11. We know about them because they have left..................
    and...

The scores for school Y were as follows :

I. ROMANS

		Per cent at each age scoring		
Age	No. of children	F and over [1]	G	B
8	14	29	0	43
9	21	33	0	57
10	30	44	3	20
11	40	62	22	25
12	34	71	18	6
13	25	68	20	20

[1] These figures include those scoring F, F+, and G.

II. Charles I

Per cent at each age scoring

Age	No. of children	F and over [1]	G	B
8	14	36	0	43
9	20	25	0	55
10	33	42	9	39
11	41	56	17	15
12	36	61	17	17
13	25	76	24	12

The papers were on the whole good. The following is one of the best. It is from the 10-year-old son of a University historian in school Y.

1. The occupations of the English were indulging in village sports, and drinking, singing, and merry-making.
2. Their food consisted of eggs, ale, and butter.
3. They lived in large country houses and their tenants in smaller cottages.
4. Their chief city was London, but during the civil war, Oxford.
5. In war their weapons were swords and blunderbusses.
6. At peace they wore velvet jackets and trousers, with lace frills.
7. On their heads they wore cocked hats.
8. On their feet they wore top boots or velvet lace slippers.
9. They worshipped Christ and to please Him they had church on Sunday.
10. Their language was Old English.
11. We know about them because they have left records of births, deaths, and marriages.

The papers marked G were about up to this standard. The same test was given at school A to children aged 10-11. The results were surprisingly bad. No one scored G, the greatest number getting F or F — on the Romans, and B on the English. The reason for this was that the answers were in a large measure identical in the two cases, and the "sandals" and "idols" fitted the Romans rather better than the English. The tests were separated by a week's

These figures include those scoring F, F +, and G.

interval, and the difference in period was carefully pointed out. The complete failure of these children in the Charles I test is all the more remarkable as they had been receiving lessons on the social life of England in the time of the Stuarts during the whole term. Practically all the children seemed to have " lumped " all historical periods together, giving them the general attributes of savagery. We could not be certain, however, whether the children failed in the test through absolute ignorance of the period or only through an inability to revive their knowledge definitely enough to put it down in writing. The next test was directed to clearing up this point.

The " pictorial identification " test

This test, given in school A to Standards II, III, IV, and V, was intended to show whether the children could recognize and distinguish different historical epochs, and, if they could, what were the indications they used in so doing. We also wished to see what means the children used to " date " the different epochs, and what knowledge they had of actual dates. For this purpose a series of three pictures was shown. All were large (about $3' \times 4'$), coloured, and historically accurate. As far as possible a definite historical event was avoided, and the scenes were those of ordinary life of the period. The pictures were :

(1) Charles I with typical Cavaliers and Roundheads.

(2) Ancient Britons.

(3) A Tournament in the time of Richard I.

In connexion with each picture the children were asked to write answers to the following questions :

I. Who do you think these people were ?
II. When did they live ? (Answer any way you like.)
III. What things in the picture tell you when they lived ?
IV. Give the name of any man or woman who was alive when these people were alive.
V. Give the date at which these people lived. Never mind if you have given it before ; give at again. If you do not know it at all, guess it, but then put " G " by your answer.

Before the test began a picture was shown as an example and the questions were answered orally by the class.

The results are best considered by taking together the answers to the same question for all three pictures, since by this means any differences due to freshness of acquaintance or to the skill of the teacher may cancel out. As the concentric method [1] of arrangement of the history syllabus is in force in this school, all the children should have learnt something of each of the periods on which they were questioned.

In answer to question I some children gave answers which were, as a matter of fact, not correct, but which could easily have been so. There was nothing in the picture to contradict such answers, though to a mind familiar with the pictures of English History, the right answer would assuredly have been suggested. For example, instead of Stuarts, French, Spanish, Roman Catholics, or " Raleigh's men " were given. Such answers were marked " vague ".

Answers such as " Romans ", " Britons ", " Danes ", or " Crusaders " to Q. I for the Charles picture, or " Romans "

---

[1] The "concentric method " is that by which the history syllabus is so arranged that the same ground is covered in successive years, but in each year the subject is treated from a different point of view, or with wider or narrower scope.

for the second, or " Danes " or " Napoleon's men " for the tournament picture were, of course, wrong.

The percentages of wrong (W), no answers (NA), vague (V), and right (R) answers to Q. I are given below.

The drop in the 12-years' results is due to the backwardness of the children tested. They would otherwise have been in a higher form. The high scores in the answers to the questions on the Britons are probably caused by the attention that is given to this period in the Elementary Schools, and also by the greater facility with which more remote periods are differentiated. As in the " completion " test, most absurdities were made in regard to the Stuarts, the period nearest and most like our own.

	Age .	8				9				10				11				12			
	No. of children	10				29				55				72				25			
		W	NA	V	R	W	NA	V	R	W	NA	V	R	W	NA	V	R	W	NA	V	R
Charles I .		50	20	20	10	24	34	28	14	31	14	31	24	29	15	36	20	28	24	24	24
Britons .		0	20	0	80	21	3	7	69	11	7	13	69	5	3	0	92	8	0	0	92
Richard I		40	10	0	50	21	38	10	31	44	14	13	29	59	6	11	33	60	8	0	32
Average %		30	16	6	46	22	25	15	38	28	11	19	40	38	8	15	48	32	10	8	47
% of W and NA		46½				47				40				36				44			
% of V and R .		53½				53				59				64				55			

The increase in the number of " vague " answers is probably due to the child's increase in scope of historical knowledge without at the same time his being able clearly to differentiate between national types. It is interesting to notice that this " vagueness " is highest at 10 years and that it decreases at 11 with an increase in correctness. This agrees well with the more positive knowledge which appeared in the other tests at this age.[1]

[1] v. Results of " Julius Cæsar " test and " completion " test, *ante*.

In answering Q. II the children chose one of four different ways of marking the period—

(a) By a date.

(b) By an epoch. This was often vague. B.C. was counted as an epoch, as were also " Stuarts ", "Stone Age", "Middle Ages ", " Olden Days ", " Days of Chivalry ".

(c) By giving the name of a person they associated with the period, e.g. " In the time of Charles I ", or " When Julius Cæsar was alive ", or " In Robin Hood's time ".

(d) By saying definitely, or indefinitely, how long ago, e.g. " 2,000 years ago ", or " a long time ago ".

The results of Q. II are shown on page 68.

On these results two questions arise, (i) what means did the children use to mark the period ? and (ii) with what degree of correctness did they use these means ?

As to (i) the most noticeable fact is the great popularity of the Date or of a Person as a time indication. Of these two the Date is the more popular at the earlier ages, but it is so frequently wrong that it cannot have much meaning. Between the ages of 9 and 10 a change occurs and the association between an epoch and a famous person of that epoch becomes the characteristic method of " dating ". Of the other two methods, " Long ago " is popular with the youngest children, but rapidly becomes rarer as they grow older. The Epoch is always rather unusual except at 10. This result may be due to accident, or it may indicate the point at which the change from the indiscriminate giving of dates is ceasing, and knowledge is hardly yet definite enough to allow them to name a Person in the period.

		8				9				10			
Age . .		8				9				10			
No. of children		10				29				55			

Percentage of children answering by :—

	D	E	M	LA	NA	D	E	M	LA	NA	D	E	M	LA	NA
Pict. I	0 *50*	10 *0*	10 *10*	20 *0*	0	3 *28*	7 *21*	7 *3*	21 *3*	10	0 *18*	7 *15*	24 *15*	14 *4*	9
„ II	10 *20*	20 *0*	0 *0*	20 *0*	30	18 *14*	14 *0*	10 *14*	7 *0*	24	27 *0*	33 *0*	4 *7*	7 *5*	18
„ III	20 *20*	10 *10*	0 *10*	0 *30*	0	13 *21*	4 *7*	14 *3*	14 *1*	25	4 *7*	11 *11*	29 *0*	4 *24*	11
Av. %	10 *30*	13 *3*	3 *7*	13 *10*	10	11 *21*	8 *9*	10 *7*	14 *1*	30	10 *8*	17 *9*	19 *7*	8 *11*	13
Incorrect + correct added	40	16	10	23	10	32	17	17	15	30	18	26	26	19	13

			11					12		
Age . .			11					12		
No. of children			72					25		

Percentage of children answering by :—

	D	E	M	LA	NA	D	E	M	LA	NA
Picture I .	3 *15*	11 *14*	20 *11*	3 *11*	6	0 *12*	4 *4*	76 *28*	4 *0*	4
„ II .	56 *0*	14 *0*	11 *3*	12 *3*	3	36 *0*	16 *4*	8 *4*	20 *4*	8
„ III .	7 *7*	11 *4*	35 *21*	4 *1*	10	0 *12*	8 *4*	28 *20*	16 *4*	8
Average % .	22 *7*	12 *6*	22 *12*	6 *5*	6	12 *8*	9 *4*	37 *17*	13 *3*	7
Incorrect + correct added	29	18	34	11	6	20	13	54	16	7

D = Date.　　E = Epoch.　　M = Man.　　LA = Long ago.　　NA = No answer.
Italic figures indicate incorrect answers.

With regard to the accuracy of the answers, there is a steady and rapid improvement in those answers which determine a Date by reference to a Person. Accuracy as regards the Date itself improves greatly between the ages of 10 and 11, but for the other ages is much the same. Accuracy as regards the Epoch is more irregular, being at its best at 10 years of age. These figures depend on the actual number who attempted to answer in these ways and do not show the comparative reliabilities of the different methods of answering. If we take the percentage of accuracy on the totals, the Date gives 47 per cent, a Person 65 per cent, and the Epoch 67 per cent. The wild use of the Date by the younger children recalls the absurd answers given in the " questions " test to the questions about the time of day by the 4- and 5-year-olds. Evidently, exact designations of time pass through a stage in which they are known, but little or no meaning is attached to them.

The answers to Q. III were interesting chiefly as showing a steady increase in ability to note definite marks of a period, and as showing that it was clothes more than anything else that attracted the children's notice.

The percentage of those who indicated definite things in their answer rose from 36 at age 8 to 72 at age 12, and the average percentage of those who noticed dress, either definitely or vaguely, was 80 as compared with 16 who noticed other things. 4 per cent gave no answer.

In Q. IV there was a steady increase in ability to give a name in connexion with a period. At 9 less than half could give any name, wrong or right, by 11 only 22 per cent failed to answer. At 9 years of age 18 per cent of the answers were right and 30 per cent wrong ; at 11, 49 per cent were right and 29 per cent wrong. The remaining percentage in either case gave no answer. It was noticeable that all the names given were those connected with battle or warfare, with the exception of King John (two children), Guenevere (one child), Wolsey (one child). Henry VIII and Charles I were also given. These have decided military connexions.

There did not seem to be any noticeable decrease in the number of guesses which children from 8 years old to 12 years old had to make in answering Q. V. The proportions who did not guess varied between 51 and 92 per cent. Dates which were not absurd were given in from 31–40 per cent of cases. There was no clear improvement with age.

The " temporal order of historical characters " test

The " picture " test gave us some idea of children's power to distinguish periods and their method of indicating a point of time by the name of some prominent person or by date. We next wished to see (i) what methods they would adopt if asked to arrange persons in sequence ; (ii) in view of their general failure in the " picture " test to manipulate dates, and the low degree of consistency achieved, whether an arrangement on a basis of dates would give the same result as an arrangement by some other means ; and (iii) what would be done in the case of people whose dates were not known.

A list of five names was therefore given to the children, and they were asked first to arrange the people in the order in which they lived, then to assign them to their proper centuries, and then to give their reasons for the original arrangement. An attempt was made to do this as a group test, but it was found unsatisfactory, and the test was then given individually. The numbers are therefore smaller, but more information was obtained. The names usually given to the children were Julius Cæsar, King Alfred, Robin Hood, Charles I, Tennyson, Admiral Beattie. They were varied according to the child's knowledge.

The reasons given by the children for their order of arrangement fell into three main types. In the case of a few of the elementary school children the people were arranged in the order in which they had entered the child's experience, e.g. " I put Robin Hood first because I heard of him in the Infant School, and I heard of King Alfred in the first form ". This type of answer was never given at school

Y. The most usual type was a rough dating by epochs, " Robin Hood lived in the time when there were few towns, he lived in the forests." In its most advanced form this type involved considerable reasoning. One boy from school Y said, " Tennyson comes late in the list. I have been reading his poems and they are not old-fashioned." A third group relied on some external means of arrangement. The simplest of these means is order in the history book. " King Arthur is before Charles because he comes earlier in our book." This can be carried over to Robin Hood, who usually does not occur in the books. " He lived about the time of William II, so he is later than Alfred."

The most advanced form of this method is the true arrangement by dates. Only one child, a girl aged 9, was found to use this method fully, though another used it in some degree. There did not seem to be any method of arrangement characteristic of a special age. The differences seemed rather to be due to greater or less knowledge of the special people given ; dates being more frequently used when the character happened to come from " our period " than when he did not. Very much the same thing occurred when a variety of the test was tried on three adults who were asked to arrange a fairly difficult list of names. It was found that a genuine historian at once assigned the names to their centuries and then put them in order. Another, who knew very little history, arranged them exclusively on the basis of epochs, though certain epochs had a vague date attached to them, e.g. Renaissance, 1400. A third, whose historical qualifications were intermediate, seemed to use a mixed system, relying on dates as far as she knew them, and then using epochs. This use of epochs in the earlier stages of knowledge is quite in accord with the greater ease of the points H, L, and E in the " Julius Cæsar " test.

When the children were asked to arrange in order by centuries the names they had already arranged in order, it became clear how little importance the majority attached to dates. This was shown in various ways. There was very little correlation between success in the two tasks. Children who had the order quite or practically right might get the dates all wrong. But more striking were the differences of order between the two arrangements. Of 14 children tested at school Y, three changed the order, although their previous arrangement was on the page before them. They did not appear to regard the second arrangement as an improvement on the other. At an elementary school, of 16 children tested aged 8 and 9, eight gave a different order with the dates. Moreover, many of the dates were quite absurd, and could only have been given if they had no meaning for the children. One boy, aged 9, who must have known St. John from scripture lessons, dated him at 1500. Another bracketed Joan of Arc and Lloyd George as both living in A.D. 300. Another gave St. John his right date, but put Robert Bruce, Robin Hood, and Charles I all earlier.

There was a general tendency to put unknown people early, which applied also to people who were known by name but with whom the children connected no period. The other well-marked tendency was to group people of the same occupation together. For example, Chaucer and Milton usually occurred in close proximity, Drake and Admiral Beattie, and on two occasions Alexander the Great and Charles I were so grouped ! This tendency is, of course, well known and widespread ; it is seen in the seven sages of Greece and in other half-legendary characters whose dates are approximated.

The " temporal memory " test

Given a reasonable understanding of the nature of time-words and relations, is it possible to show that time-marks possess less significance for children than other details, and disproportionately less for children than adults ? Certainly adult forgetfulness for such details as the time of a meeting is very marked, and children seem to be even more unreliable. We used two tests for an investigation of this point. The first was the reproduction of a story that contained details of various kinds, the object being to see if one type of detail was forgotten more readily than another. The second was the composition of a letter asking a friend to come out for a walk, the aim here being to see if the children would remember to name both the time and place of meeting, or would forget one more often than the other. In the memory test various stories were used, the two main ones being *Archbishop John* and *Chenklo*. In all cases the story was read through once, and the children were asked to reproduce it in writing after an interval of from 20 to 30 minutes. They were told in advance that this reproduction would be required. In marking, the stories were split up into what seemed separate ideas, and these were counted as correct even if the wording was not exactly right, or if they were displaced from their proper place in the story. The " inaccuracy " of the memory of any point was taken as the percentage of times the point was wrongly remembered in proportion to the total number of times it was remembered at all. This percentage is later called the coefficient of inaccuracy.

     A   B   C   D

Archbishop John | was a patron of art | in Denmark. | In the summer |

  E   F   G   H

of 1679 | 3 | poor boys | came to ask him to help them to learn painting. |

        I   J   K   L

They arrived on Sunday | morning | at his palace | at Copenhagen, |

        M   N   O

and said they had walked | 152 miles to see him. | The servant | said the

        P   Q   R

Archbishop would be busy all day. | They must come again | at 6 o'clock

     R_1 S

in the evening. | They amused themselves in the public gardens | which

        T

were only 100 yards | away till the Archbishop could see them. | He

      U   V   W

gave them each £27 | and made them stay in the city | during the month

          X   Y

of June, | to see the great works of art | preserved in the churches there. |

  Z   *a*   *β*   *γ*   δ

In after years | two of them, | William | and Martin, | became painters

                ε

famous | throughout Europe. |

     1   2   3   4

Chenklo | was a brigand | who lived in a cave | on a rock | which

   5   6   7

towered 1,120 ft. | above the Caspian Sea. | He was only 48 | but his hair

        8   9

was already as white as snow. | 17 devoted followers | were ever at

    10   11

his beck and call. | The cave was stored with gold and jewels, | but he

      12   13

became ever sadder and more silent. | Twice a year, | once when the

      14   15

first swallow returned, | once on the 8th of November, | he retired to the

       16   17   18

topmost peak of the mountain | and spent two days | in lonely

         19   20   21

meditation. | None knew his secret, | but in his last years | he retired to a

            22

monastery | and became a devoted servant of the Church. |

It could not be expected that the time details, however unimportant they might be, would all be found together at the bottom of the list. With stories of this nature various circumstances may affect the position of the different points, e.g. a certain romantic interest seemed to attach to Chenklo's hair being white, and this probably affected the number of individuals who remembered his age. In another test, the results of which were closely similar (and which are therefore not given), an age not connected with any

POINTS ARRANGED IN ORDER OF DIFFICULTY, BEGINNING WITH THE EASIEST.

Archbishop John

I. 18 children, 12–14

No.	Point	Percentage remembering it correctly	Coefficient of in-accuracy
G	Poor boys	78	0
A	Archbishop John . . .	72	23
H	Ask him for help . . .	72	0
O	The servant told them . .	72	0
δ	Became famous painters .	61	0
P	Archbishop busy . . .	61	0
F	3	56	33
U	Gave each £27 . . .	50	25
R	**At 6 o'clock in evening** .	39	0
S	*Public gardens* . . .	39	21
a	Two of them . . .	39	0
C	*In Denmark*	33	0
L	*At Copenhagen* . . .	33	0
M	They had walked . . .	33	0
T	100 *yards*	33	33
V	*In that city*	33	0
γ	Martin	33	0
I	**Sunday**	28	0
Z	**In after years** . . .	28	0
ε	*Throughout Europe* . .	22	0
N	152 *miles*	22	50
B	Patron of art . . .	22	77
D	**In summer** . . .	17	57
J	**Morning**	17	0
W	**Month of June** . . .	17	0
K	*At his palace* . . .	17	0
X	Great works of art . .	17	0
E	**1679**	11	71
Y	*In the churches* . . .	11	0
β	William	11	71
Q	They must come again . .	6	0

Time in heavy type.   Place in italics.

II. 20 adults

No.	Point	Percentage remembering it correctly	Coefficient of inaccuracy
δ	Famous painters . . .	95	0
C	*In Denmark*	80	0
G	Poor boys	75	12
M	They had walked . . .	70	0
α	Two of them . . .	65	13
U	Gave each £27 . . .	65	7
B	Patron of art . . .	65	19
H	Ask him for help . . .	60	0
A	Archbishop John . . .	60	37
O	Servant told them. . .	55	26
F	3	50	50
γ	Martin	40	20
S	*Public gardens* . .	35	36
P	The Archbishop busy . .	35	36
L	*At Copenhagen* . . .	35	12
E	**1679**	35	50
Q	They must come again . .	30	0
β	William	30	33
J	**Morning**	25	0
K	*At his palace* . . .	25	0
X	Works of art . . .	25	16
Z	**In after years** . . .	25	16
R	**6 o'clock in the evening** .	20	0
T	100 *yards*	20	20
W	**Month of June** . . .	15	50
N	152 *miles*	15	80
Y	*In the churches* . . .	10	50
ε	*Throughout Europe* . .	10	33
D	**In the summer** . . .	10	0
I	**Sunday**	10	0
V	*In that city*	5	0

Time in heavy type.　Place in italics.

POINTS IN ORDER OF DIFFICULTY

Chenklo

I. 73 children

No.	Point	Percentage remembering it correctly	Coefficient of inaccuracy
3	*Lived in a cave* . . .	84	0
11	Cave full of gold . . .	81	2
8	Hair as white as snow . .	73	0
16	*Went to peak of mountain* .	66	6
7	**Only 48**	64	18
6	*Caspian Sea* . . .	60	15
12	Grew sadder. . . .	53	2
21	Retired to a monastery .	49	18

No.	Point	Percentage remembering it correctly	Coefficient of inaccuracy
2	He was a brigand . .	41	14
9	17 devoted followers . .	41	47
17	**For 2 days** . . .	40	12
22	Servant of the church . .	33	27
13	**Twice a year** . . .	31	18
19	None knew his secret . .	30	19
10	Followers at his call . .	29	5
4	*On a rock*	26	14
18	In lonely meditation . .	25	0
20	**In his last years** . .	18	53
14	**When the swallow returned**	14	50
1	Chenklo	11	87
15	**8th November** . . .	10	59
5	1,120 ft.	8	88

Time in heavy type.   Place in italics.

II.   8 adults

No.	Point	Percentage remembering it correctly	Coefficient of inaccuracy
9	17 followers	88	0
2	Was a brigand . . .	75	0
11	Cave full of gold . . .	75	0
12	Grew sadder	75	0
13	**Twice a year** . . .	75	0
16	*Peak of mountain* . . .	75	0
21	Retired to a monastery .	75	0
3	*Lived in a cave* . . .	63	0
19	None knew his secret . .	63	0
4	*On a rock*	50	0
7	**He was 48**	50	43
8	Hair as white as snow . .	50	0
14	**When the swallow returned**	50	43
15	**8th November** . . .	50	43
22	Servant of church . .	50	20
1	Chenklo	32	50
5	1,120 *ft.*	32	53
6	*Caspian sea*	32	0
10	Followers at beck and call .	32	0
20	**In his last years** . .	32	40
17	**Spent 2 days** . . .	25	0
18	In lonely meditation . .	12	0

Time in heavy type.   Place in italics.

such detail came out bottom. Moreover, some points are more closely connected with the fabric of the story than others, e.g. the first five points in *Archbishop John* could hardly have been missed without destroying the story. But allowing for these causes of irregularity, it can be seen from the tables that the details of time and space do form a sediment, as it were, at the bottom of the lists, and that of these two time holds a lower place than space. The percentage of people remembering correctly the different types of points is :—

		Time	Space	Others
Ch.	Children	35·4	48·8	43·3
A. J.	Children	23·1	27	45·5
A. J.	Adults	20	26	54·6
Ch.	Adults	47	50·4	55·2

It can be seen that space has always a superiority over time, and that both space and time are, except in one case, inferior to the other points taken together. In this one case it seems that the slight superiority of space is due to the fascination for children of " life in a cave ", which heads the list.

The tables of the inaccuracy coefficients show that it is not to time or place as such that inaccuracy mainly attaches, but to all definite names and figures. With few exceptions, all the high coefficients (over 20 per cent) belong to names or figures. In two of these cases, " patron of art " and " servant of the church ", the mistakes were due to a failure to understand the phrases. The other three are marks of time : " in his last years," " in summer," and " the first swallow," and may perhaps be due to inattention to time. However, the numbers who remembered the existence of these points were small. In spite of the inaccuracy in recall, we do not find a sediment of names and figures at the bottom of the lists as we do with time and place. The mistakes in many cases suggest that it was the effort to recall the details *exactly* that proved difficult. The figures were represented by some vague phrase, "some poor boys" taking the place of " three ", or " one day " taking the place of " in summer ". It was not rare to get an " about " added to the round number, e.g. " about 1,100 ft.", as if the writer were rebuking the experimenter for being unnecessarily precise.

From this test, then, we can get some experimental evidence of the observed fact that time details are remembered with more difficulty than others, but the evidence does not show that this inability to remember is more marked in children of ages 12–14, the ages tested, than in adults. Such inability would probably have been shown more clearly if we had used younger children, but the difficulty of using the same tests on both groups would then have been too great. If, as was suggested above, time-knowledge begins to assume its adult form at about 11, this would account for the result.

The last test was intended to illustrate the same point, when the problem was not one of memory but the formation of plans of future action.

The "making an appointment" test

This test gave much more definite results. The instructions to the children were : " Write a letter to a friend arranging to go out for a walk with him." The letters were mostly quite short, and the greater number made a definite appointment to meet. In these cases it was possible to see how many gave both time and place of meeting, and how many forgot one or the other. Of 153 children of various ages tested, 128 gave a definite place of meeting, only 84 gave a definite time. Of the others, however, most gave an indefinite or inadequate time, e.g. to-morrow, or Tuesday afternoon. Very few gave absolutely no time indication at all. There is a slight improvement with age up to about 13. Owing to the conditions of the test, the 14-year-olds were more stupid than the others. The numbers at 11 years of age are too small to be reliable.

| | | Per cent giving | | |
Age	No. of children	Time	Place	Difference place-time
8	12	33	92	59
9	23	61	87	26
10	25	60	88	28
11	7	86	71	– 15
12	32	72	94	22
13	32	59	66	7
14	22	59	87	28

Some children gave both time and place.

From these letters it seems possible to imagine how the plan presented itself to the children. In one case they thought of a vacant afternoon to fill, and the letters read, " Can you come for a walk on Saturday afternoon ? " In others the object of the walk was more prominently in mind, " Can you come for a walk to Leigh Woods ? " Of the two the latter was the more likely to lead to the making of a definite appointment ; in the former the writer seemed apt to give no further time-indication, apparently feeling that what was so clear to him must be equally clear to his friend. We can conclude, then, that in forming plans time is less important to children than space, and that the tendency is very strong for a vague time to take the place of a definite one.

A child in a community which has developed a system of time-indications and a framework of conventional time, naturally starts with a great advantage over a tribe which is forming these designations for itself. The child does not have to invent words or concepts, but merely to learn the use of the terms which it finds current. A further difference is introduced because a child learns at once the more abstract terminology, and is discouraged from using the more concrete designations which appear natural to the savage, e.g. the child finds that numbers are the customary designa-tion of days or years and is not encouraged to refer to a year as " the time when I did so and so ". Yet, in spite of this, such a designation is frequent.

Bearing this in mind, the relation between the individual learning of the time scheme and the development of it by the race is sufficiently striking. A child, like a savage, has a very limited outlook. He is concerned with the matters immediately before him, and the time periods that he knows are of frequent recurrence, and are known concretely. For example, in the " questions " test the part of the day was first known, then the day of the week, then the month, the season, the year, and lastly the day of the month. This order in the growth of knowledge is supported by the absurdity tests. When the children were asked for reasons for thinking it was morning or July the answers they gave were always concrete and referred in the one case generally to their own meals and in the other to natural phenomena, exactly as many primitive peoples distinguish the periods of the day by actions, and nearly all distinguish the seasons by differences of vegetation or weather.

The month seems to present the same difficulties to children as it does to savages. The modern child is cut off from the savage resource of observing the moon as an aid to distinguishing the days of the month, and he seems to share the savage's objection to counting, especially to counting time units. He naturally finds it hard to remember the days of the month, just as very few primitive peoples have arrived at the stage of numbering the days right through the month. This difficulty of remembering the day of the month does not, unfortunately, end in childhood, but continues to adult life, and makes most men the slaves of their calendars.

One other difficulty common to children and savages does seem to vanish with age, that is the inability to understand the year. At a certain stage primitive peoples seem to arrive at the idea of a year, just as children appear to grasp its nature at a definite point in their development. Somewhere between 6.5 and 7.5 children become able to give the date of the year. From the other experiments it seems very unlikely that they know what this date means, but the mere fact of being able to give a date shows that a question relating to the year has some meaning. At this stage children are in a position similar to savages who recognize years as we know them, but do not organize them into an epoch. A child recognizes the year as a unit, calls it by the number which is its common designation, but does not recognize that the number is one of a series arranged on a special principle. The nature of the series is grasped some 3 or 4 years later, just as a numbered series of years with an era is a comparatively late and rare invention among the races of the world.

Except in those tribes which keep records of past years, any event of more than a few years ago is apt to be referred vaguely to the " past ". This is also characteristic of children's thought. Unless they have been very well taught, or come from educated homes, historical periods are all " lumped " together and generally given the characteristics of the most remote. There is no organization of the past. If a thing is not present, or so nearly present as to seem almost within personal experience, it may have happened any time. Granny, aged 80, may easily have known Robin Hood. This point has been referred to before, and will be dealt with again in the discussion of the manner in which past and future are arranged as a series.

There can, I think, be little doubt that, as an organized experience, space precedes time. A savage can find his way about, even makes long voyages, when he is still unable to tell the time accurately. So, with children, apparently, time bulks less largely in their exact thought than space. We can compare with this some of the dreams of adults which show a similar contrast between the precision of the indications of space and time. In my own dream records, and in the dream of others, it is no uncommon experience to find the account illustrated by a plan, not only of the actual things seen, but of parts of the house and landscape which were invisible to the dreamer. Time indications, on the other hand, unless the dream scene included some special mark, e.g. " a sunset sky ", are very rare.

I have left the matter of duration till the end, because it is the subject of the next chapter. It is noticeable that questions on it come low on the list in the first test, and it is certainly one of the aspects of time which caused most difficulty in the organization of the calendar. The psychological reasons for this may be clearer later.

CHAPTER V

DURATION

WE have seen that measures of duration are invented late and that most children have considerable difficulty in learning to use these measures. This is partly due, in the case of the shorter measures, e.g. minutes and seconds, to lack of practice in their use ; it is also due, with both longer and shorter measures of time, to subjective variations of experience.

In ordinary life we can make passable estimates of duration ; it is only when we attempt a fairly high degree of accuracy that we notice our insufficiencies. We can generally tell approximately when we have done a morning's work, and, if a friend promises to meet us in half-an-hour, and keeps his word, we are not generally surprised by his returning much sooner or much later than we expected. On the other hand, if we try to estimate 30 minutes exactly there are very likely to be considerable errors in our estimate, errors which render such an estimate unfit for use in a co-operative society. Even without exact measurements it is common experience that time appears to vary in length according to the nature of the events which occupy it or the state of mind in which we are ; and this experience naturally raises the question of how we estimate duration. It is necessary, however, first to discuss the *nature* of the experience of duration.

It was said in Chapter II that events must be assumed to have a certain temporal extension. This means that experience, at any moment, is not narrowed to a point, but that a specious present, as William James named it, exists. Whether this character of temporal extensity is capable of any further analysis seems doubtful. It does not, however, form more than a part, and perhaps not a very large part, of the experience of duration as we know it in ordinary life. For example, suppose we are asked to estimate the period of time during which a pencil is held up, we can note in addition to the mere experience of temporal extension (a) the consciousness of a number of mental events, thoughts, images, which pass through the mind ; (b) a certain amount of fatigue of attention or of the eye muscles ; (c) certain changes in the external environment. All these changes are easy to observe, and their variations can be definitely associated with the length of time to be estimated. But they are not the whole of the experience of duration, as we can see from certain contrasting experiences in which we have the element of change and extensity separated. The best example of change without the experience of temporal extension is a dead faint. One moment we are standing up, the next, apparently, we are on the floor. There is change, but no time seems to intervene between the beginning and the end of the faint. In fact, the lack of the ordinary time spacing of events is the most interesting feature of the experience. A converse experience throws into prominence the extension factor, when there is, consciously, the minimum of change. It often happens in games, feats of skill, or in solving problems that we become so absorbed in our occupa-

tion that conscious reflection practically disappears. An
oarsman in a race may hear the starting gun, and then find
that he is rowing the *second* stroke. A child walking on a
wall may balance desperately at a difficult bit—and find
himself safely over it. In neither case is there any definite
consciousness of what happened during the short period of
rowing the first stroke or regaining the balance, but the
interval does not drop out as in a faint. On the contrary,
it presents a peculiar quality of great duration, quite
divorced from the ordinary measures of time. We must
then see in the experience of duration these two factors,
extensity and observed change; the one, extensity, really
lying at the basis of the whole experience, since a succession
of discontinuous changes, such as are experienced in a faint,
would not give us anything like the idea of time we
possess to-day; while the other, change, as I hope to show
later, becomes increasingly important when we attempt to
estimate duration; since it obviously varies with different
lengths of time.

Before we can estimate duration, we are faced with another
difficulty : in terms of what is the duration to be estimated ?
Duration is essentially a subjective experience, and is thus
contrasted with the experience of simultaneity which is
concerned with external happenings. Of this subjective
experience we have no convenient measure naturally given ;
it is no easy task to devise one.

The early difficulty in estimating or representing duration
is the absence of a unit. Considered from the subjective
standpoint there *is* no unit. How can one compare, from the
point of view of experienced duration, the length of a

night's sleep, a spell of work, or an unhappy interview with the dentist ? This is probably the reason why, when units were invented, periods of the night were for so long reckoned in different units from those of the day. It also explains the primitive preference for counting time by simultaneity rather than by duration.

The difficulty was solved by externalizing duration. It was reckoned not in subjective units of experience, but in movements of external objects, in fact it was reckoned very much as equal times are defined in mechanics to-day, by reference to the spaces through which equal bodies pass under similar circumstances. Actually to-day time is defined by the " pendulum " which, by an escapement, has its ticks measured off on a wheel and communicated to a dial ; but, before this was arranged, many semi-exact methods were tried, such as hour glasses or graduated candles, or time was reckoned in terms of space travelled, the time taken to boil a cauldron of vegetables, or to " go to the market and buy a water-melon ".[1]

The tendency to externalize any duration that has to be estimated is as strong as ever to-day. The ordinary person when asked to estimate a short time adopts a method which is essentially the same. He counts the period in what he believes to be seconds, or swings his hand in the manner of a pendulum. This preference is amply justified by experience. With a suitable method of tapping, far greater accuracy can be attained than with estimates made without its aid, and, in certain experiments I made, the error was between three and four times as great when the subjects simply estimated the time as when they counted in taps.

[1] Cf. " Hassan ", Flecker.

This obvious fact, that it is far easier and more usual to judge the length of time intervals in reference to some regular physical event, has led Münsterberg and others to declare that all estimates of short times are based on conscious or unconscious counting of, e.g. heartbeats, or breathing. This contention has not been supported by further experiment,[1] and, as far as introspection serves me, I believe that it is quite possible to form estimates of time without using any kind of counting. It is this direct estimate of time which is subject to such great variations, and which, indeed, often appears to be absent—generally absent with small children, provokingly absent on certain occasions with adults.

The estimates of duration seem to depend on a certain division of attention, we both experience and reflect on the succession of experiences ; and if this division of attention is destroyed, as when we become excitedly immersed in some occupation, we are apt to become oblivious of the passage of time. This failure of the time estimate seems to occur also in moments of emotion, whether pleasant or unpleasant. I have had instances of it reported to me as occurring during a bombardment, a concert, and very acute toothache, and in all cases the expression was the same : " You lost all sense of time, and could not tell afterwards whether it had lasted hours or minutes." [2] A variation of this experience is given in the following account of a day's fighting.[3]

[1] R. S. Woodworth, *Psychology* (1922), p. 439.
[2] Cf. James Thompson, *Insomnia*, st. vi.
[3] Privately communicated by W. Freeman, R. Sussex Regiment.

" About one month after my introduction to front-line work on the Somme, in 1916, my battalion was ordered to assault the famous Schwaben Redoubt. As this was to be my first experience of going ' over the top ', it would be pardonable and no exaggeration to describe my feelings as out of the normal. My particular company was composed of fresh and untried young men of Kitchener's Army, as keen as possible to distinguish themselves, full of ' esprit de corps ' and, alas, inexperience. I mention this to show that the prevailing feeling of my comrades and myself was excitement—the excitement, if you like, of the chase. This particular attack was timed for about 9 a.m. one morning, and was preceded by a terrific bombardment, which, as it worked up to maximum intensity, was met by a counter barrage from the enemy. All this turmoil—for the earth rocked like the sea in a storm—had the effect on our untried men of stringing them up to a still further pitch of excitement. The signal given, we dashed from what had been trenches towards the enemy's lines, from which, after a struggle, he was dislodged. In our impetuosity we somewhat overran our objective. This necessitated a halt, and the process of ' digging ourselves in ' to consolidate the gains won. This last is one of the most arduous technical tasks of the infantry man. But the extraordinary part of this experience—one quite apart from the novelty of tasting war at first hand—was the trick my senses seemed to play me with respect to time.

" From the signal of our officers to charge until the close of the preliminary work of digging in, at the going down of the sun on that October day, the operation appeared to me to last, say half-an-hour—nay, perhaps hardly so much. The sun seemed literally to move visibly in its semi-circle from horizon to horizon. As excitement died down, and normal self-control and appraisement resumed its sway, this curious delusion—if it was one from a scientific standpoint—was forced upon my notice, and has remained one of my most striking memories of the Great War."

A similar illusion occurs frequently on waking suddenly from a deep sleep at some unusual time. One is quite unable to estimate the time one has been asleep, and the first tendency is to assume that it is morning. A sleeper roused after only a few minutes' sleep will ask if it is time to get up. I have wakened at 3 a.m. in October and guessed that it was 6 a.m., misinterpreting, in my sleepy condition, moon-set for sunrise. Occasionally, the belief that it is morning is so strong as to produce an optical illusion. A Scotch woman (a student) of very regular habits was accustomed to wake by an alarm clock and call the servant. She had been working late in bed, and went to sleep at midnight. She woke, thought the clock had failed to go off, struck a match, and looked at it and saw that it was just past seven. She called the servant and put the kettle on and went back to bed, and began working again. Presently the servant came in giggling. " What time do you think it is, miss ? " " About 7.45." " No miss, quarter to two." And when she looked at her clock again she saw it was so.

In all these cases the illusion appears to be due to the simple absence of *real* material on which to base the estimate leading to a misinterpretation of such indications as are given from without. Similarly, in ordinary working life, the people who are most liable to " forget the time " are generally those who possess most power of absorbing themselves in an idea or conversation.

A certain amount of attention, therefore, needs to be given to the passage of time, as such, if it is to be estimated, and the following factors are usually mentioned as affecting this estimate. (a) The number of events occurring in the period to be estimated,[1] (b) the pleasantness or unpleasantness of the experience,[1] (c) the amount of attention devoted to time, as such, during the period.[2] In the ordinary course of events it is assumed that the greater the number of events, the longer the period appears, the greater the pleasantness the shorter, and the more attention devoted to time, as such, the longer. When we get pleasantness and a large number of events combined, as in William James' example of a period of travel, the events are assumed to pass quickly but to appear long in retrospect ; vice versa, a period of unpleasant dullness is long to experience and short to look back on.

So long as these different methods of judging time are all being employed, or could all be employed, as they are, or could be in any of our ordinary estimates of time, it is exceedingly difficult to assign the right degree of influence to each of them. There have been very few experiments directed to discovering the effects on time estimates of variations in the manner in which the time is spent, and of these few some have fallen into an error in relation to the use of the term " number of events ", or similar phrases. It

---

[1] W. James, *Textbook of Psychology*, ch. xvii.
[2] Romanes, *Consciousness of Time, in Mind*, 1878.

appears from William James' account, and from others also, that " event " is taken primarily in the sense of external event. In discussing estimates of time such a restriction is a mistake. "Event" should be used in the sense of mental event, and mean any sensation, thought, or emotion, of which we are conscious, whether this "event" comes from outside or is of mental origin only. But this of course introduces a new difficulty ; while it is possible to control the external events and produce a " filled " or " empty " interval at will, it is very hard to control, and harder still to register, the flow of " mental events " which pass in the subject's head.

It is easier to control the pleasantness or unpleasantness of the filling of a time interval; and the following experiments were undertaken with the intention of investigating this factor in time estimates : although, as will be seen, the results are actually more concerned with the first of the factors mentioned.[1]

As all the estimates were made as part of time experiments, the amount of attention devoted to the passage of time, as such, was practically constant.

The plan of the experiments was simple. The subject was asked (a) to estimate, in terms of seconds or minutes, the time that a pencil was held up, or (b), in some series, to start a stop-watch and to stop it when a certain number of seconds had elapsed   Some lack of precision was involved in method (a) ; but as the times used in this experiment were comparatively long, this was not serious. Three series of experiments were undertaken : (1) a trial series in which M and N acted alternately as subject and experimenter, and method (a) was used ; (2) a series con-

[1] The following experiments were originally published in the B. J. of Psy.

ducted by the writer alone, using method (b) ; and (3) one in which the writer was subject and O experimenter, both methods of procedure being used. The times varied from one or two seconds to one minute.

In all three series of experiments the effects of practice were, so far as possible, guarded against. In (1) neither subject knew her own results, though the course of the experiment naturally familiarized her with the different periods. In (2) no special precautions could be taken as the writer was working alone. In (3) the subject had no knowledge at all of her results and was not using the stop-watch for any other purpose at the time.

In all cases the estimates of time were made in sets of from six to eight estimates on each occasion. For each set two measures were calculated : (i) the average percentage error, irrespective of sign, (ii) the percentage ratio of the estimates as a whole to the actual time. Of these two measures (i) shows the general correctness of the series, (ii) shows whether the time as a whole appeared too long or too short, the ratio of course being larger than 100 in the former case and smaller in the latter.

Experiment 1. The results obtained from subject N show considerable irregularity both as regards accuracy and the comparative length of the real and apparent time. There is no constant tendency to judge the times as either too long or too short ; and there is no sign of improvement with practice.

A larger number of sittings were obtained from subject M—in all 15 spread over 16 days. The results were similar to those from N, except that the irregularities are greater, the average error varying from 60·8 per cent (series 2) to 6·4 per cent (series 1) and the ratio from 153 through all degrees to 58. As in *N's* results, there is no definite practice effect discernible.

Towards the end of this series of experiments the effect of pain on the time estimate was studied. At the beginning of a sitting the subject started to smoke, and whenever the experimenter raised the pencil she brought the lighted end of the cigarette against her hand, keeping it there till the pencil was lowered. The following table gives the results for that sitting (No. xii) and for the four sittings which preceded and followed it in the experiment; the latter were carried out under approximately the same conditions except for the pain.

TABLE I : Subject *M*

No. of sitting	x	xi	xii	xiii	xiv
Average percentage error	22·7	33	19·4	36	42·5
No. of estimates with + error	6	2	3	0	1
No. of estimates with − error	3	5	3	7	7
No. of estimates correct	0	0	1	0	0
Percentage ratio to actual time	105	96	98	68	74

The result is interesting and was quite unexpected. Of the five sets here given, xii (the pain series) has the smallest error and the percentage ratio is nearest to 100. It contains also the only quite correct estimate in the five series. Taking the results of the whole experiment for *M*, xii is the fourth best as regards average error, and the percentage ratio is nearest to 100 in the whole series. It is therefore one of the best sets of estimates, and in it the estimated time shows least definite bias in either direction.

Experiment 2. The circumstances in which this series of experiments was conducted were intentionally very varied. The series falls into three groups—(*a*) comfort, (*b*) discomfort, (*c*) in the railway train, which are *not* mutually exclusive. The conditions considered comfortable were—(*a*) in bed at night before settling down to go to sleep, (*b*) in a room alone during the day, (*c*) in the train when the experimenter was in a compartment which was quiet and sufficiently airy. Discomfort included (*a*) the prick of a pin, (*b*) considerable hunger when waiting for a meal, and (*c*) a stuffy railway carriage with a screaming baby in it. It will be observed that the experiments performed in the train include conditions both of comfort and discomfort. In certain of the experiments under comfortable conditions, an attempt was made to fix the attention by listening to (without counting) the ticking of a clock in the room. In all, 32 sets of estimates were made, the experiment lasting over 12 days. On many occasions more than one set of estimates was made at a sitting, the subject leaving only long enough between the sets to prevent fatigue or to make changes in the conditions. Except in special cases the subject allowed her thoughts to wander. When the experiments were carried out in the train she usually looked out of the window.

Dividing the results into three groups—Comfort, Discomfort, and Train—they are as follows :

TABLE II

	Total No. of series	Average percentage error	Percentage ratio of estimated to actual time
Comfort	16 (excluding those in train)	25·6	91
Discomfort	7 ,, ,,	24·4	89
Train	9	28·7	106

The Comfort and Discomfort results are practically identical, the tendency being for the subject to find time pass too quickly. The results for experiments done in the train are markedly different. The average error is rather larger, and the ratio shows that the subject found the time too long. That this result is not due to feelings of comfort or discomfort is shown by the fact that the train series included conditions of both kinds, and also by the results of certain comfort and discomfort series which were expressly arranged to be closely parallel to each other, and in which the results were practically identical.

Subjectively the distinguishing mark of the train experience was that the subject was continually entertained with the scenery or the movements of her fellow travellers. On the other occasions when carrying out the experiments she was alone, and though her thoughts wandered, they did so without much external provocation.

In some of the experiments, as stated above, the subject attempted to keep her thoughts fixed on the ticking of a clock. This was always done under comfortable circumstances and the series was made parallel to other comfortable series, during which the mind was allowed to wander. The results of comparing five series when the attention was thus fixed with five parallel ones when it was not are :

TABLE III

	Average percentage error	No. of cases			Percentage ratio of estimated to actual time
		with + error	with − error	correct	
Attention fixed	26·7	19	6	5	79
Attention free	26	13	13	4	85

In these results the average error is approximately the same ; but the ratio is lower in the series with the attention fixed, thus showing that the time seemed shorter. Now the subject had a strong objection to these experiments. They were distinctly more boring than usual and the attempt to attend to the ticking and so exclude irrelevant thoughts involved an unpleasant effort. At the same time, in so far as this attempt was successful, the " amount of thought " during the interval of time was decreased.

The extreme percentage ratios are : " Attention fixed " = 79, " In the train " = 106 ; while the ratios for Attention Free, Comfort and Discomfort series are intermediate. This means that time seemed shortest when there was least range of mental activity, longest in the train when there was most, and intermediate in other circumstances. The pleasantness or unpleasantness of the experience seemed to have little effect.

Experiment 3. In the interval between this and the pre-ceding experiment, the writer had worked out the results of experiment 2, but on a basis quite different from that given above. She did not, therefore, start the following experi-ment with any definite theory prejudicing her mind.

Two sets of experiments were now carried out each day, one in the morning about 10.30, the other in the evening about 11 o'clock. The morning experiment consisted of three series—(1) the procedure being as in experiment 1, (2) with procedure as in experiment 2 except for the fact that the subject did not record her own times, (3) as in (2) except that the subject was reading aloud from a book (a translation of Gogol's *Taras Bulba*) throughout the whole experiment. In the evening two sets were performed—1a and 2a—the procedure being the same as for (1) and (2) above, except that the subject was always smoking.

The results are as follows :

TABLE IV

Morning Experiments. Subject M

Series	A	B	C	D	E	Av. of all series
Average percentage error :						
Series 1	25·5	33·3	24·7	35·1	34·3	30·5
2	17	39·8	43·8	33	63·6	39·4
3	19	31·1	37·1	18	43	29·6
Percentage ratio of estimated to actual time :						
Series 1	83	67	75	65	66	71
2	83	73	65	69	45	67
3	111	108	111	94	58	96

In these results the average error is approximately the same for series 1 and 3. It is highest for series 2. This shows that the grave distraction incident to reading aloud had no prejudicial effect on the power to estimate time. The ratios, on the other hand, show that reading increased the apparent length of time. The whole tendency in these experiments was to judge time too short. The result of reading is to make the estimated time approximately the same as the real time.

These results are in accord with those of experiment 2. There the movement of the train made the time seem long ; here reading, with its consequent production of ideas, has the same effect.

The evening experiments were intended to test once again the effect of pain on estimates of time. As in experiment 1, the pain was a fairly severe burn from a lighted cigarette. In the following table the pain series is K.

As in the morning experiments, the procedure of 2a give larger errors than that of 1a, but the difference is not so marked. The ratios are closely similar, the time always appearing shorter than in reality.

TABLE V

Evening Experiments. Subject M

Series	F	G	H	K	M	Av. of all series
Average percentage errors :						
Series 1a	39	16	30·6	38	20·6	28·8
2a	21·5	23·6	16	41·6	59·5	32·4
Percentage ratio of estimated to actual time :						
Series 1a	61	94	100	62	79	79·2
2a	97	91	84	58	40	75

The pain series—K—is distinguished by having the second largest error in the series, but this error is always in the same sense—negative. The times, therefore, appeared much too short. In fact, the ratio for this series is almost the lowest (cf. experiment 1) in the whole research. This apparent shortening of the time seems to be due to a fixation of the attention comparable to, but more extreme than, that in the series when the subject listened to a clock ticking. The pain series in experiment 1 bears the note : " I think I did these estimates well, as my attention was fixed."

Chance providing an opportunity in an acute attack of earache, an attempt was made to carry these experiments on to the estimation of longer periods. The subject M attempted to estimate an interval of five minutes, using method (b). As no experiments of this kind had been done for many months, the subject made one estimate overnight to get an approximate standard, and then the four estimates given below next morning. The ratio of estimated to actual time were

128, 111, 107, 110

In all cases the time appeared slightly longer than reality. For similar estimates made under normal circumstances, compare page 117, where the times give ratios of from 128-105. The estimate of Time, therefore, even for somewhat longer periods, does not seem to be altered by discomfort.

These experiments, then, confirm the statement that in estimating time we rely on the amount of mental content experienced during that time, and are against those who find the determining factor of the estimate in pleasure or displeasure. Time which has been filled by many thoughts appears longer, whereas time occupied by few thoughts appears shorter. In particular, time spent in the train or in reading seems longer, time when the attention is immobilized by a ticking clock, or yet more forcibly by pain, seems shorter. On one occasion in the morning series of experiment 3, the subject felt that she had given unusually correct estimates. Her mind was clear and empty ; no irrelevant ideas intruded, and the idea of time was kept clearly before the mind. This series was E 2. It will be seen (Table IV) that the error is the largest in the series, and the ratio the smallest. Thus on this occasion time passed at its fastest for that experiment.

A crucial case is that of waiting for a friend who fails to keep his appointment. The generally accepted analysis of the situation is that one has nothing to do, therefore the experience is unpleasant, and therefore it seems long. The time undoubtedly seems long and the experience is unpleasant, but it is not certain that these facts are causally connected. The unpleasant feeling tone may be due to a thwarted conation. We long to be away to our destination, to begin our talk. Our pride is hurt by being thus kept waiting through another's carelessness ; we are worried lest we shall miss our train or get no supper. The apparent length of time seems to have another cause. So far are our minds from being at rest and unoccupied, that they are a very frenzy of whirling thoughts. They swarm with words of reproach, with anxious speculations as to the cause of delay, with plans for the future, etc. We will not let ourselves read, but turn the pages of the books on the nearest bookstall, trying by the greatest possible number of stimulations to distract our minds––and so we increase the time of our torment ! The apparent length of time spent in waiting is due rather to the number of impressions we force upon ourselves than to the unpleasantness of the experience.

This principle, that apparent length of time depends on the amount of mental content, is also in accordance with general experience. A period of travel may seem long in experience as well as in retrospect. Twenty-four hours which the writer spent in Paris seemed, and seem, about the length of an ordinary week ; and it was a pleasant experience. On the other hand, days of joy when the attention is focused on a single beloved object fly past. The case of a woman— a sufferer from insomnia—is quoted by Binet,[1] whose fear of not getting her five hours' sleep made the nights apparently pass in a flash. We can also explain on the same

---

[1] *Arch. de Psychol.*, 1903.

basis Janet's [1] observation that years seem to pass more quickly with increasing age. In old age, it takes longer to arrive at an idea, longer to act than in youth. Therefore the years actually hold less for the old. This is an easier explanation than Janet's own, and perhaps better than James's.[2]

With this theory regarding time estimates we may compare two well-known facts : (a) when a person is asked to estimate the relative length of two historical periods— e.g. if asked which was the longest time, from the first invasion of England by the Romans to the Norman Conquest or from the Norman Conquest to the present day— he is likely to judge that period to be the longer about which he knows the most. Abundance of content will give the impression that the time is long ; (b) the illusion of filled and empty space. Here in the realm of vision we have the same principle—if a space is filled it appears larger than one which is empty.

The farther question naturally arises as to whether the apparent length of a period depends directly on the number of mental events which occur during the period, or whether it is estimated in some other more complicated way. This point can hardly be made the subject of exact investigation, as we can scarcely control the flitting thoughts of any subject, however conscientiously he concentrates on some particular object ; but it is possible to use a metronome as a rough test of the effect of a differing number of external impressions. If estimates are made when a metronome is

---

[1] *Rev. philos.*, vol. iii.
[2] *Principles of Psychology*, ch. xv.

set ticking 40 to the minute, and then when it is ticking at 208, the time should, in the latter case, appear five times as long as in the former, supposing always that there is an exact correspondence between the number of events and the time estimate. The results of experiments show no such effects, because every subject knows that in one case the ticking is at a greater rate than in the other, and makes allowances accordingly. What actually happened was that time seemed a little longer with the fast ticking ; the ratios being (av. of 10 subjects, 3 estimations each) 134·6 with the slow ticking, 147·3 with the fast.

One subject in this experiment (his results are excluded above) illustrates a danger which attaches to all these experiments on duration—the tendency for estimates to be affected by all sorts of (experimentally) irrelevant factors. This subject is a calm person, quite free from any nervous excitability. He was the only one of the subjects who did not find the time too long and who did not complain of the noise the metronome made. His ratio for the slow ticking was 72 and for the fast 24. When asked for introspections, he said, " The slow is irregular and no help in judging, and the fast ?—I kept saying to myself, ' the damned thing is trying to hurry me, but *I'll resist it.*' " In this he was so successful that when asked to give a time of 35 seconds, he gave two minutes three seconds.

It is possible that it is not only the number but the disconnectedness of mental events which affects the judgment of duration. If we are thinking about a single topic, a number of ideas, all relevant to that topic, do not seem to produce a lengthening of the time similar to that produced by a number of disconnected events or ideas. A rough example of the effects on the sense of time of continual distraction is afforded by a ride on the top of a London bus. My own experience is that time estimates under those circumstances are extremely unreliable, and that time appears very long. It is only a definite knowledge of the time a ride takes which enables me to form any idea of its duration.

There is one set of facts which appears to be contradictory to the above, that is the power to wake from sleep at a given hour. Many people claim to be able to do this with great accuracy, but the definite experimental results are scanty.

Tschisch has made observations on himself and Vaschide [1] has conducted experiments on himself and 33 other subjects.

Tschisch notes that his error in waking rarely exceeds 15 minutes, and is on the average 13 minutes, and he always wakes earlier than the hour named.

Vaschide is primarily concerned with proving that the attention is active during sleep, and that the fixation of the attention on the hour of waking affects the character of the sleep. He states that only three out of his subjects found that they slept absolutely normally under the particular circumstances, and that in two subjects, specially studied during the night before waking at a set time, the pulse rate was above that of the subject in ordinary sleep, and that there were marked signs of disturbance, increasing as the time of waking drew near.

As regards the power to waken at a fixed hour, he found considerable variations with sex, age, time of year, and other

[1] *Le sommeil et les rêves*, ch. iii (1911).

factors. The average error for his subjects was 21 minutes. One subject in seven experiments had errors which varied from 4 minutes to 37 seconds. On the other hand, one young woman was quite incapable of waking herself, and woke as much as 1 hour 25 minutes late. On the whole, the subjects woke early (28 early to 5 late), and woke more easily in summer than at other seasons. The younger found it harder to wake than did the elder, and the subjects who had had little or no education woke more exactly than the educated. Thirteen highly educated persons had an average error of 25 minutes with large individual differences. Those with a rudimentary education (6) had an average of 12 minutes 30 seconds, and three subjects with no education gave an average of 7 seconds with very small individual variations. Vaschide farther finds that the accuracy of waking increases as the time set approaches the normal waking time of the subject. If, however, it is later, the error tends to increase greatly. This, however, is not so with all subjects. Vaschide's subjects were specially chosen for their powers of waking, and when I have attempted to repeat the experiments I have been keenly conscious of my inferior powers. My experiments fall into three groups. A. I attempted to wake, with no intention of getting up, at 4 a.m. B. The time set was 6 a.m. I again did not get up, but just looked at my watch. C. The time set was 8 a.m. I had a particular reason for waking at that hour, and had to get up then. The results of the series show marked differences. In A the average error is 17 minutes 30 seconds. I only woke once—near the time set—and then went to sleep again. In B I woke up too early and dozed and woke

until approximately the right time when I allowed myself
to fall asleep. The average error for the first waking was
2 hours 20 minutes, and on one occasion I woke four times
before 6 o'clock. In C on many occasions I woke much too
early at first, and then a second time before the hour. The
average error for the first waking was 1 hour 5 minutes. The
largest error was 1 hour 30 minutes, the smallest 2 minutes.

The explanation of the comparative success of series A
is that I naturally wake, if I am going to wake in the night,
between 3 and 4 a.m. so that the time set coincided fairly
well with my normal time of waking. The other results
give little indication of any estimate of duration, or, if such
an estimate is formed, it is extremely unreliable. I appear
rather to be determined to wake, and to go on waking un-
easily till I achieve approximate success. Vaschide's results
also, though far better, show no particular indication of being
due to a judgment of *duration* ; in fact, certain points which
he notices in connexion with them are in favour of a different
explanation.

Vaschide notes (i) that it is easier to wake to time in
summer than in winter. In summer there are more indications from light, sun, etc., as to the time. He says (ii) that
people wake more exactly according as the time set
approaches their normal waking time. Certain bodily
sensations of hunger, thirst, etc., probably co-operate in
waking them. Then again (iii) the less educated subjects,
who were probably more accustomed to judging time by
natural signs, woke better than the highly educated who
habitually relied on watches. Moreover, Vaschide notes
(iv) that persons attempting to wake at a certain hour

showed during sleep signs of excitement which did not
occur on other occasions, and that this excitement increased
as the hour of waking drew nearer. The sleeper clearly has
his attention occupied, and this increasing excitement is
more natural if he is attending to external indications,
which more and more clearly approach the state antici-
pated, than if he is merely making an estimate which would
involve no progressive excitement.

Farther, as we all know, the plan generally adopted by
one who wishes to wake early is to fix the hour of waking
firmly in mind, and not to calculate the distance in time
between the hour of going to bed and the time set for getting
up. Moreover, experiments of Professor Boring's [1] have
shown that it is possible to make a very good estimate of
the time of waking by relying on such " cues as the feelings
of fatigue or restedness, which indicated the duration of
sleep, of inertness or the degree of sleepiness, which indicated the depth of sleep, and bodily cues such as the course
of the excretory and digestive functions."

The truth of the matter is probably contained in the old
fairy tale. A princess on a journey once changed clothes
with her maid to prevent her identity being discovered.
On their way they took refuge in a castle. The
knight who owned it being attracted by the seeming
maid wished to decide which was which, and asked the
princess and the maid the following question : " How do
you know when to get up in the morning ? " " Oh," said
the disguised princess, " in the morning the ring which I

[1] *Studies in Psychology. Titchener Commemorative Volume* (Cornell).

wear on my finger turns cold, and then I know it is time."
The maid, who was dressed as the princess, replied, " At
home when I milk the cows in the morning I always take a
drink of the new milk, so, when I begin to feel thirsty, I
know it is time to get up and have my drink." These
answers left the knight in little doubt as to the identity of
his visitors.

CHAPTER VI

DURATION (Continued)

THOUGH the estimate of duration depends largely on the number of events which occur during a period, that is not, I think, the sole criterion employed. There is a very common illusion which suggests that another factor is involved in time estimation. It has frequently been noted that long dreams, appearing to last some hours, may occur in a few minutes or seconds.

An extreme example of this type of illusion is afforded by the dream of the Marquis de Lavalette, which occurred while he was in prison during the Terror. It occupied the few moments during which midnight was striking and the guard outside his door was being changed. The dream runs as follows (I have somewhat abbreviated it) :

" I was in the Rue Saint Honoré. It was dark and the streets were deserted, but soon a diffused dull murmur was heard. Suddenly a troop of horsemen appeared at the end of the street . . . terrible beings, bearing torches . . . For *five hours* they passed me by, riding at full gallop. After them came a vast number of gun carriages loaded with dead bodies. . . ." [1]

This illusion occurs in many cases, but not in so striking a form. The main difficulty in studying dreams of this type is to discover the maximum time within which the dream occurred. When we know this, we know that the dream

---

[1] Quoted by Tobolowska, *Des illusions du temps dans les rêves du someil normal.*

cannot have taken longer than a certain time, and so we have some measure of this illusion. Occasionally it is possible to determine the time, as in the dream given above, or in the following dream, which the dreamer kindly told me.

" When I was demonstrator in a physiological laboratory I found it hard to wake in the mornings. One day my father came up with a bell and rung it once—up and down—so that it gave two strokes. I dreamed that I was ready to lecture and rang the bell for the body to be brought in. I gave my lecture and dissected an arm, and rang for the body to be removed. The dream occurred between the two strokes of the bell."

On occasions, I have observed the total length of sleep in which a dream has occurred, but in these cases the time given includes falling asleep and waking, and the exact length of the dream is therefore uncertain.

N. dozing before getting up in the morning. Total time of sleep eight minutes. The dream ran :

" You and I have been all round a Mentally Deficient School. We have watched the children, talked to the head, and discussed Blake with him (only it was really Fra Angelico). We were quite leisurely over it. We spent the whole afternoon there." Again N., dozing in the afternoon. Total time of sleep six minutes. She woke saying, " I've been having such a lot of dreams and doing so many things." The dream reported was, " I was on an expedition which came to a river which had to be crossed ; we made preparations for crossing, some stuck in the mud and struggled ; and a lot of other things happened."

Attempts have been made to show that dreams are instantaneous, and the argument is generally based on dreams which lead up to, and terminate in, some striking event which is clearly connected with an external stimulus, e.g. a dream of the French Revolution ends on the scaffold, and the dreamer wakes suddenly to find that the rail at the head of his bed has fallen across his neck.[1] It is then supposed that these dreams are really constructed backwards, i.e. the falling bar, which appears on the end of the dream, really starts it ; and the preceding part of the dream is a rationalization of this event, and is thought of between the bar touching the sleeper and his apparently instantaneous awakening.   So firmly has this theory taken root that articles have been written explaining exactly how this remarkable mental feat can be accomplished.[2]   However, there seems not the slightest reason for supposing that dreams conform to this theory.   In the first place not all external events thus weave themselves into the tissue of our dreams.   We are far more often wakened out of a dream by some incongruous event than enabled to incorporate that event in our dream.   Secondly, to accept the speed of dreams demanded by this theory is to render mental processes in sleep little short of miraculous ; and Du Prel,[3] in his discussion of these dreams, boldly forsakes man and invokes God.   Thirdly, there is a certain amount of evidence from dreams themselves that they are not instantaneous, since external events which occur at certain intervals appear, when they form part of a dream, as separated by a

---

[1] Maury, *Le sommeil et les rêves.*
[2] Histon, *Journal of Abnormal Psychology*, 1916–17, p. 48.
[3] *Philosophy of Mysticism*, ch. iii, § 1.

certain time, though the dream time may not be the same as the actual. The following is a dream of N.'s.

" I was giving a demonstration lesson, and all through it there was a low hum. I tried to locate it in the class, but I couldn't, and I went on talking. I seemed to get through quite a lot of material, although I can't remember what it was. . . . At last I found one child in the back row was humming on one note. I stopped her, and she laughed. I woke up, and at once noticed the ship's sirens, which I can hear. Each boom lasts about 10 seconds at longest. I realized at once what the noise in the dream had been."

A dream of L.'s.

L. and her father and his friend went out for a walk together. The friend wanted to shoot pigeons, and L. and her father went on in advance to pick up the birds. Bang ! he shot, and the bullets went whizzing past their ears. They looked for birds but found none. Bang ! he shot again, and the shot went rather higher, but still dangerously near. They went on looking for birds. He shot a third time, Bang ! right over the top of a thorn bush. Then they went on their walk.

In this dream the bangs seemed a long time apart, about half an hour, perhaps. The dream occurred just at the time to get up, and there were three bangs outside the house at this time, but they were not in reality more than two seconds apart.

I have attempted to do some experiments connected with this time spacing of external events in dreams. My results are scanty owing to the difficulty (a) of being sure that the subject is asleep and not merely lying quiet, (b) of giving a stimulus which would affect her dream without waking her. The stimulus which was found most satisfactory was a slow pressure on the wrist or hand. A touch on the face always woke the subject. The pressure was considered hard enough when the subject moved. Here are two comparatively successful attempts. Subject N.

I took her wrist and pinched it till she moved. Then waited 5 breathings (she woke if I clicked my stop-watch) and pinched the wrist again. I woke her at once and asked if she had been dreaming. She was sleepy, and answered, " I was climbing down the rocks at G. and ropy seaweed kept lashing out and catching round my ancle and wrist." I asked, " How often did it happen ? " " Every time you put out your hand so (showed with right hand, the one I had pinched) it caught."

In this dream a double pinch is represented by a plurality of " catchings ", but the number is not well defined. In the second experiment only a single pinch was given, and in the corresponding dream it is represented by a single contact on the hand.

Subject N. I took her wrist and pinched it as before, and woke her about three seconds afterwards. She said, " I was dreaming that I was falling over the cliffs at C., then a tree caught my hand, and then I was falling, and something caught my knee. . ." In my own case I have woken from a dream of workmen hammering to find the blind flapping at just the same rate.

These observations indicate that dreams have sufficient duration to allow of the representation of events separated by a certain interval of time ; there is no need to imagine for them any mystic quality of instantaneousness ; nor, further, is it necessary to imagine that the rate of thought in them greatly exceeds that of waking life. Many of the dreams which appear to contain many events, and which are judged as occupying a long time, seem on reflexion to have very little content. In the dream of the dissection, the dreamer stated that really his lecture had no content. In a dream of my own, which occurred in a four minutes' doze, I was taking a Latin class. One child asked me a question about the parts of *fio*, and then "there was a general feeling of much questioning by the class. I thought ' I am managing this lesson badly as I am so sleepy to-day '." The dream appeared to be the length of an ordinary lesson, but the dream content was extremely scanty. In a similar way, if a person talks in his sleep, only a few words, or a disconnected phrase or two, may be uttered ; yet the dreamer asserts on waking that he has carried on quite a long conversation. It is quite possible, therefore, that the content of dreams is often far less than the record of them would lead us to imagine, even though in some of them the speed of thought may be greater than that of ordinary waking life.

We can attempt to estimate the rate of thought during waking life by allowing a series of images to pass through our minds for a set period, e.g. 10 seconds, and then recording the series.

Supposing we attempt to form a series of visual images or to think of a number of events, the record of thoughts during a period of ten seconds may run something like this.

Subject C. (a rowing man). " Went down to barge ; sat about ; coach did not come. At last coach was seen crossing

over from Merton barge to towpath. Got into boat and
pushed off.   Then we rowed a bad first stroke and paddled
down to the Gut." This would make the record of quite
a fairly long dream ; yet when the subject guessed the period
which had elapsed, he thought it was four seconds.   In
experiments on myself the record of images during ten
seconds is rather shorter, but would still make a fair dream.
The same holds good for other subjects, and, in all cases,
the time occupied was estimated as too short ; usually under
half of the actual time. From this last fact it would appear, if
we may assume that estimates of time do depend mainly on
the number of mental events, that the rate of this thinking
" to order " is slower than the normal.   It seems, therefore, that in most of the cases there is time for the events
of a dream to be thought of, without presupposing any
marvellous increase in the rate of thought.   There is, moreover, another point.   It is possible that some types of
thought and imagery may be speedier than others.   In
waking life most people have so definite a preference for
one form of imagery that it is difficult to get really comparable records of thought when using other types of imagery.
In my own case a very noticeable change takes place with
oncoming sleep.   In ordinary waking life my imagery is
almost entirely kinæsthetic-verbal, but, just before falling
asleep, visual imagery predominates.   I therefore made time
estimates under three conditions in order to see if there were
any noticeable differences.   I attempted to estimate the
time by starting my stop-watch and stopping it when I
thought that a period of five minutes had elapsed.   In all
cases when I performed the experiments, I was lying down

with intent to go to sleep. In the series called A. I was so sleepy that my imagery was visual; in B. I was fairly sleepy, but still thinking in words ; C. I was also fairly sleepy, but was telling myself some story or other. I made eight estimates in each series, and they were made on different occasions and in such an order as would distribute the effect of practice equally among the series. In all the series I tended to stop the watch too soon ; i.e. time appeared longer than it really was. This was most marked in series A., least in C., and B. was nearer to C. than A. The percentage ratios for the apparent to real time were :

Series A. 128·4 visual,
,, B. 110 verbal,
,, C. 105·2 story.

It seems likely from these results, that thought which takes place in visual images is slightly more rapid than thought which uses other types of imagery, and, as dreams are predominantly visual, this may account in part for their greater speed.

For all these reasons, then, we cannot explain the time illusions of dreams as due to the greater number of mental events which occur during the period. It seems rather that we make a judgment of the *nature* of these events, that this judgment is false, and produces the illusion. Dreams occur when we are physically still, and they possess hallucinatory vividness. We seem to be acting, and yet there is no movement. In waking life the necessity of physical movement is a continual drag on the speed of our thought. An action as simple as starting and stopping a stop-watch takes from o·6″–1·8″, and, whilst this is being done, our thought is limited to the action, and the speed of thought is accordingly decreased. The consequence is that, in active life, we assume that so many events occupy a certain amount of clock-time. When we know we are only thinking of actions, and not performing them—as in the image formation experiments above—we expect a much greater number of events to be contained in a certain space of clock-time. In dreams there is a speed of actionless thought combined with the belief that we are acting, and then the judgment as to the amount of clock-time occupied by a series of events is at fault.

A very similar condition and illusion is found in the visions of the drowning. These visions seem to occur at the moment when struggling has ceased and physical movement is at an end. They are also characterized by hallucinatory vividness, and seem to occupy a time far greater than they actually do by the clock. The following abbreviated account, which is typical of many others, illustrates these points.

A young man aged 20 was bathing with a friend. He was swimming under water when his friend dived in and accidentally struck him, driving the air from his lungs, and he sank to the bottom of the river. He lay quite still and, though conscious that he was drowning, made no effort to save himself. The events of his life passed slowly before his eyes. He saw his funeral and heard the stones rattle down on his coffin. He heard the bells ring, saw many coloured pictures. He felt a peculiarly vivid sensation of comfort, and imagined that he was floating off from earth to heaven. He then appears to have lost consciousness and to have recovered through his friend's ministrations.[1]

This theory of the estimate of duration, that it depends on a judgment of the number and the nature of mental events which occur in a certain period of conventional time, demands that we shall have a fairly good memory for time durations and a certain faculty for dividing them, e.g. we need to have in our heads a scheme which allows us to estimate whether the events we have experienced would fill an hour or half an hour. For the different periods what we normally use, each of us arrives at a very fair estimate. Most lecturers of any experience know how long the material they have prepared will last, and a teacher prepares for a 35-, 45-, or 60-minute lesson with a clear idea of the differences in their time values. In other professions other periods are schematized. The photographer can guess five seconds with considerable accuracy, and the oarsman has a good idea of the speed of his stroke. Some people seem singularly skilful at such estimates. The following are some results from a boy of 16 years whose only previous practice had been a game of guessing 3-minute periods, played as a means of beguiling the tedium of Latin lessons.

The subject had a stop-watch, which he started and stopped after the required time had elapsed. The experimenter read the times. When he gave one time and doubled it he did not know the length of time originally given. The interval between the original time and the second estimate was about 2 minutes. He was asked not to count as an aid to his estimates, and said he did not do so.

[1] Quoted by Tobolowska, op. cit.

I.

Time aimed at	1 min.	1'	30"	30"	19"	12"	5"	30"
Time given	57 sec.	57·4"	28"	32"	19"	13"	5·8"	30·2"

II. Asked to give a time and then the half of it.

Time given	17·4"	1' 39"	10"
Half	8"	49"	5·4"

III.

Original time	11"	doubled to	20·4"
,, ,,	13"	⅓ given as	4"
,, ,,	5·8" × 3	,,	16"
,, ,,	24"	$\frac{1}{10}$,,	3"
,, ,,	2" × 10	,,	21·5"

In II and III the subject nearly always had in mind the length of time he was aiming at in his first period, so that these results show a power to estimate conventional time rather than to divide periods of experienced duration.

As a contrast, the following results illustrate the powers of estimating short periods of time possessed by the average person. In this case the subjects did not aim at any definite length of conventional time, but were attempting to judge experienced duration directly ; they were not told the length of their original times.

Subject X. Method as before.

Original time	1' 44"	repeated as	1' 51"
,, ,,	36·8"	,, ,,	42·5"
,, ,,	22"	½ given as	25"
,, ,,	52"	,, ,,	36"

Subject Y.

Original time	21"	repeated as	36"
,, ,,	53·6"	,, ,,	40"
,, ,,	31·5"	½ given as	21·5"
,, ,,	48"	,, ,,	17·5"

These two subjects, though both highly educated, were quite unpractised, and had no reason to be familiar with periods of time shorter than a minute.

The nature of these results shows that there is a fair memory for the experience of duration even when it is not related to a time scheme, and that, when connected with a conventional time scheme, a very high degree of accuracy can be obtained. There is, therefore, no absurdity in supposing that ordinary estimates of duration involve a comparison of experienced duration with an ideal scheme. The uncertainty of the estimates are just what might be expected in such a comparison.

In consequence, perhaps, of the uncertainty of our own judgment of duration, we have been ready to tolerate great irregularities in the representation of it, especially on the stage. At some periods of the drama the unity of time has been insisted on, and the dramatic time has been expected to coincide with the actual time; at others the most barefaced devices have sufficed to represent hours or centuries. Johnson, in his preface to *Shakespeare*, states :—" Time is, of all modes of existence, most obsequious to the imagination ; a lapse of years is as easily conceived as a passage of hours. In contemplation we easily contract the time of real actions, and therefore willingly permit it to be contracted when we only see their imitation."

In many of Shakespeare's plays the time order of the scenes is uncertain. Some scenes, as happens in the *Merchant of Venice*, being in reality simultaneous, though successive in representation ; other plays allow long and undefined periods to elapse between the scenes. In this, Shakespeare is in the direct tradition from the morality plays in which a turn about the stage served to bridge the space of time which lay between Adam and Noah. Marlow's *Tamburlaine* uses this licence more freely than Shakespeare. In its extreme form the licence is nowhere better illustrated than in the Thibetan plays translated by Bacot and Woolf, where both time and space are completely conventionalized, and cause no more trouble in the play than they would do in an Epic poem.

The modern convention is halfway between the licence of this tradition and the temporal severity of the classicists. The whole dramatic action need not fall within the three hours' space of the play, but the dramatic and real time of the different acts must coincide. Where the programme mentions a lapse of time there it may occur, not otherwise. One of the criticisms of the recent production of *Hassan* commented unfavourably on the short time occupied by the torture " off ", though we were given to understand that Rafi and Pervaneh suffered a *lingering* death.

This refusal to allow the imagination to rule time indicates a growing consciousness of duration in relation to conventional time marks. It shows that though we may still frequently misjudge time, we have a more firmly organized time scheme in our minds than had our ancestors of some few generations ago.

CHAPTER VII

ORDER OF EVENTS IN TIME

IN a previous chapter it has been suggested that the distinction of the past, present, and future arose through a combination of memory and purpose ; and that in its early stages this distinction was not accompanied by any definite ordering of the events of the past, or an exact anticipation of the sequence in which the future would occur.

With little children to-day much the same thing seems to happen. Quite early a distinction appears between the immediate and the remote past, and perhaps between the immediate and the more distant future ; but in the records of children's speech or answers there is little to suggest that they are able to arrange events, past or to come, in a definite series. On the other hand, most adults make such an arrangement, or at least can make it when called on to do so. The means by which such an arrangement is made are far from clear. Mention is usually made of " movements of attention " or of " fading brain-states " in any discussion of this point, but little is said of any process of construction or reasoning, witting or unwitting. It will perhaps be worth while to examine two typical forms of these theories.

Professor James Ward makes the distinction of past, present, and future depend on the waxing and waning of images from the central point of the vivid present, and combines this with a theory of the " movements of attention " to account for the existence of order in the past. These movements of attention constitute for him the " temporal signs " by which experience is arranged. " Thus," he says, " psychologically regarded, the distinction of past and future seems to be identical with the two facts just described. It depends, that is to say, (1) upon the continuous sinking of the primary memory—images on the one side, and the continuous rising of the ordinary images on the other side, of that member of a series of percepts then repeating which is actual at the moment : and (2) on the prevenient adjustments of attention, to which such words as ' expect ', ' await ', ' anticipate ', all testify by their etymology. . . ." [1]

Within the past, order is established under the following conditions. " The first condition of such awareness is that we should have represented together presentations that were in the first instance attended to separately. This we have in the persistence of primary memory-images and in the (comparatively) simultaneous reproduction of longer or shorter portions of the memory-train constituting the pre-perceptions or expectations that the actual present normally entails. In a series thus secured there may be time marks, though no time, and by these marks the series will be distinguished from other simultaneous series ; these we may call the second condition.

" To ask which is first among a number of simultaneous presentations is unmeaning ; one might be logically prior to another, but in time they are together and priority is

[1] *Psychological Principles*, p. 211.

excluded. Nevertheless, with each distinct representation
a, b, c, d there is probably connected some trace of that
movement of attention of which we are aware in passing
from one presentation to another. . . . These residua are
our temporal signs, and, together with the representations
connected with them, constitute the memory-continuum.

" But temporal signs alone will not furnish all the pictorial
exactness of time perspective. They give us only a fixed
series ; but the working of obliviscence by ensuring a progressive variation in intensity and distinctness as we pass
from one member of the series to the next, yields the effect
which we call time distance ; this we may call the third
condition.

" By themselves such variations would leave us liable to
confound more vivid representations in the distance with
fainter ones nearer the present, but from this mistake the
temporal signs save us ; and, as a matter of fact, where the
memory-train is imperfect such mistakes continually occur.
On the other hand, where these variations are slight and
imperceptible, though the memory continuum preserves
the order of events intact, we have still no such distinct
appreciation of comparative distance in time as we have
nearer the present, where these perspective events are
considerable." [1]

I have quoted this account somewhat in full because it
is a careful combination of a theory of temporal signs with
one based on the varying force of memory, and is an obvious
improvement on such an one as Fouillée's, which depends
entirely on the varying degrees of clearness of the memory
of different events.

[1] Op. cit., p. 214.

" On each side of the present stretches a series of gradually increasing desire and gradually weakening memory . . .
The establishment of order in a series of events is achieved
by event C, at maximal intensity, being connected with B at
second intensity, and A at third. The three representations,
being fused together into a single whole by coenæsthesia,
etc., when we are given C, B, and A, are recalled in order
of clearness." [1]

This theory is included in Professor Ward's, so that both
can be criticized together on this point. There can be little
doubt that Fouillée and Professor Ward are definitely
wrong so far as they attempt to explain the arrangement of
time on the basis of relative clearness of memory. When we
think of a series of just-past events, e.g. a day spent in town,
we do not start from an event C at maximum memory
intensity (the walk home from the station) and then connect
B (the return train journey) with that, and with that again
A (securing a corner-seat at Paddington), and so on backward
from one event to another of ever less intensity and greater
remoteness. On the contrary, we either think of the most
outstanding feature of the day—a visit to Wembley ; or,
if we wish to go through the events of the whole day, we
start at the beginning— our early breakfast—and " so draw
to a conclusion ". The type of remembering, which Fouillée
describes, does occur in one class of memories, and it is
sufficiently different from our ordinary experience to call
for special notice. In recalling dreams we tend to remember
backwards in the manner which Fouillée describes. In a
charming record of dreams [2] the following advice is given to

---

[1] Fouillée, *Psych. des idées-forcés*, p. 101.
[2] Arnold-Forster, *Studies in Dreams*, p. 79.

the would-be recorder. " In recording, the dream should
first be allowed to unroll itself very quietly *backwards* in a
series of slowly moving pictures, starting from the end and
going back slowly through scene after scene to its beginning
until the whole dream has been seen." The value of this
advice can be tested any morning when waking from a rather
confused dream, and the peculiarity of this type of memory
and of the time order noticed. We only use this type of
memory when trying to recall our waking deeds on the
occasions when our acts have been particularly disorganized ;
on the other hand, we abandon it when recalling a particularly vivid and well-constructed dream.

Fouillée's theory is open to another objection, which is
noticed by Professor Ward. Events at a distance may be
more vivid, owing to their character or importance, than those
which have occurred more recently. If we judged the order
of events simply by the intensity of the memory, confusions
of this sort would be almost certain to occur. They do
occur, but less frequently than would be expected if this
criterion of vividness was the only one employed. This
argument applies not only to the past, but also to the future.
It is not always the immediate future which is the most
vivid. My most intense desire at the moment concerns a
week-end visit a fortnight away. The events of the intervening time interest me but little, and the nearest event—
going to bed—interests me not at all. I have practically
no desire to go. Unfortunately the greater force of desire
does not bring the week-end any nearer actually or mentally,
nor am I in any danger of confusing the probable order of
events.

The additions which Professor Ward makes to the theory of decreasing vividness are open to somewhat the same objections. The movements of attention, which he postulates, and their traces would most naturally lead to a reverse order of presentation, as in the case of the vividness theory. If it does not, the two principles of arrangement are at variance with each other and it seems difficult to see how a compromise is arrived at. Moreover, with events at all remote, it is impossible to detect any trace of the movements of attention ; and, as we have seen above, any past beyond the immediate tends to lose its order and become a mere mass from which items are taken as need arises. Even in cases of fairly recent memory the certainty of the time order is far less than Professor Ward would lead us to suppose. In a simple experiment an attempt was made to test the accuracy of the memory for serial order in matter which had little internal principle of arrangement.

Four poems [1] were chosen which were likely to be unknown to a class of students. They were read out without comment, and the class was told not to think about them if possible. The next day the students were asked to write down the titles of the poems (or as much as would make the subject clear) *in the order in which they had been read.* (Results A.) Two days later they were asked for a second reproduction of the titles. This second request was apparently quite unexpected. (Results B.) They were also asked to give the means by which they had remembered the order of the poems. These introspections were only given in quite a

[1] They were, " The Black Greyhound," " Days too short," "An Example," " Storm," on pp. 243, 135, 136, and 391 of J. C. Squire's *Anthology of Modern Verse.*

few cases and are often meagre, as the class was unpractised in introspection; but they show the most general and obvious methods of arrangement adopted.

No. of Students—27.

A.

No. of papers correct, 5.
,,   incorrect, 22.

Distribution of poems as read and reproduced, incorrect papers.

	No. as written	1	2	3	4	omitted.
	1	18	1	1	0	2
No. in order as read.	2	2	9	5	2	4
	3		7	2	2	11
	4			6	9	7

Mean contingency, ·487.
Correlation (about), ·88.

B.

No of papers correct, 6.
,,   incorrect, 21.

Distribution of incorrect papers.

	No. as written.	1	2	3	4	omitted.
	1	19	2			
No. as read.	2	1	11	6	1	2
	3		5	4		12
	4			3	15	3

Mean contingency, ·570.
Correlation (about), ·93.

These results show that it is by no means universal for disconnected events presented in a serial order to be remembered in that order. The arrangement involves as definite an act of memory as do the items to be arranged. In a few of the introspections an indication is given of the methods by which this arrangement is made :

(*a*) (from an incorrect paper) " The subjects were alternately black and white—black greyhound, sun, darkness of storm, then light again." In this case the last two poems were transposed to make them fit into the scheme.

(*b*) (an incomplete paper, No. 3 omitted). " By a visionary imagination—by placing mind-pictures in the order in which they were formed,

$$\text{thus} \quad 1 \quad 2$$
$$3 \quad 4."$$

(*c*) (a correct paper) " First was about animals, second nature, third nature, fourth elements."

From this it is clear that in many cases the memory of the order depended on the witting invention of some connecting idea or formulation, or, in the case of visualizers, on an arrangement of mental images. In my own case, when learning the order of the poems, the most noticeable feature was the rapid formation of a language habit in saying the short titles by which I distinguished them.

These results are supported by certain experiments on remembering the order of a series of picture post cards shown once to the subject. The subjects were asked to give the cards in the order in which they were shown, and were then asked to describe each and to say which they liked best. Most subjects remembered one of the five better than the others, and some had definite preferences, but there did not appear any tendency to put the one best remembered, or preferred, last in order, although there were many mistakes in reproducing the arrangement.

It is thus clear that, whatever method we use in remembering the order of events, it is by no means infallible ; and that, when it is unusually difficult to give the order of events, some special aid is often wittingly adopted, and that this aid is not connected with either movements of attention or with the relative clearness of the different memory traces. On the contrary, clearness of memory does not seem to enter as a factor into the arrangement of the time order ; and movements of attention, if they contribute to it at all, do so in a very minor degree and only when events are very recent.

At the same time a serial arrangement is habitually made of the events of waking life, and we can gather some idea of the peculiar nature of this arrangement when we contrast it with the cases in which no temporal order of experience appears, or in which the time arrangement seems to be based on a different principle. The dreams in my collection which illustrate this point fall into four groups.

(1) In dreams there is sometimes a definite simultaneity of apparently incompatible activities. In one dream the dreamer was arranging a college syllabus and talking to people in the room and doing the two things not successively but simultaneously. This simultaneous character of different trains of thought seems to occur on certain occasions in waking life. One informant tells me that she never thinks of the reasons for and against a theory in succession, but all together. I have also heard moments of philosophic insight described in which the whole question seems to " open up

together ". We can also compare the oft quoted case of Mozart, saying that he could hear all his music " together ".

It is then quite possible to have a number of mental events presented not successively, but simultaneously— without a time order. There is therefore no reason to suppose that a time order is always given, though we very seldom apprehend any set of events without one.

(2) Events may not stretch out in a definite chain, but be implied by one particular event. " On Friday night I dreamt that I was at the theatre box-office trying to get seats for *What Every Woman Knows*. There were no upper circle seats, only 12s. 6d. ones (said the man) in the stalls. I considered getting them, and gradually (fairly quickly it seems) mother and I were sitting in the stalls watching the play. It was the evening, with the sense of all the day's happenings between Saturday morning and Saturday night quite clear and definite. The problem was one I was facing in waking life ; but, in the dream, time had slipped on—the wish, or imagined situation, came true at once with the sense of intervening happenings *as part of* the one event."

(3) In opposition to this telescoping of time we more often get a time insertion containing the past. This seems to be a fairly common mode of time presentation in dreams. I will quote one example. " You and I were in a tram with a large, tall, muscular man with a beautiful voice. . . . We got off together—and he said he was going on—if he may. We talked of him, and suddenly in the second of time in my dream I lived over again all my previous experiences with him. We had met on a seat while waiting

for a 'bus. I had asked him the time—to seem friendly, and we had become close friends from that moment. We— all three of us—had driven in a motor-car, and had tea at a lovely old inn. All this was not mere reminiscence, it *was* experience, familiar yet fresh, and it was lived in the space between two sentences in conversation. It was explanatory and *actual*. I mean I enjoyed the ride and felt the air and tasted the tea again—yet not again, but freshly as if for the first time."

This insertion of time has an interesting parallel in an old English fairy story,[1] in which the Noon Fairy gives to a youth a bag of Time's sand which, if held in the hand, gave extra time to the holder unexperienced by the rest of the world. A bag of 60 grains held in the hand would give an hour inserted between e.g. 11.59 and 12 o'clock, and no one would perceive it except the holder of the minutes.

The other element in the dream, the re-experiencing of previous experience, introduces a further interesting complication into this type of time experience, and seems most akin to the revival of emotion when a subject under hypnosis is asked to relate some experience in the past.

(4) Lastly, there are dream experiences in which time is simply reversed. " I dreamed a dream backwards last night—even to the extent of falling uphill ! I fell up a steep slope with all the sensations of falling down— and then proceeded to live from effect to cause. It was not very clear, but I was in bed, then I was on a 'bus coming home, then I was crossing a road, dodging traffic to catch

[1] *Faery Gold* (Everyman's Lib.), p. 269.

a 'bus—and so on. . . . I seemed to be living that way, perfectly normally."

It is possible to imagine yet other variations of the time order, but I will not discuss them now as I have not examples of them in actual experience. Those that have been given are enough to show that the method of arrangement actually adopted in memory is by no means inevitable or the only possible one. It seems rather that it is the result of different factors and is constructed by the aid of various forms of reasoning.

It will be convenient to divide the cases to be considered into two groups, (a) those in which we actually remember the order in itself, and (b) those in which the order is definitely a matter of inference based on dates or other associations. The cases under (a) are mostly of a fairly recent date ; those under (b) concern more remote memories, though the method may also be used with recent memories.

If we look back over a period of time which has just ended, say our activities during a morning between 9—1, we do not at once recollect them all or recollect them in a time order. This is particularly striking if the period has been occupied by a series of " odd jobs ". One thinks of this or that event or action in itself, but not as connected temporarily with other events. If it is desired to arrange the events in a time order, the procedure is something as follows. " I played with the kitten, yes, that was at 11.0, because I had him with me when I was drinking my coffee. I invigilated ; that was just before, because I did it from 10.30 till 11.0. Then I was at a meeting ; that must have been after I played with the kitten, as I went straight from the meeting to a lecture at 11.30, and I did not take the kitten to the meeting though I wanted to." Thus the separate items are arranged. The arrangement within any particular item is of a different sort. Take the item of the lecture. I collected my papers, crossed to the lecture building, went straight upstairs, and reflected that I could not be bothered to fetch my gown as it was late, went along a corridor, went into the room, and waited for the chattering to stop, looked at my papers, and found that I had the wrong notes—decided that it did not matter, as I could lecture from memory, and so on.

In the first case, the events are arranged in order by means of conventional time marks and reasoning, in the second by reference to a scheme of purpose, cause and effect, and to some extent to space. Our memories, like our actions, are organized around certain purposes, and, as our actions succeed one another in relation to these ends, so can we follow our memories step by step. Guyau noted this fact clearly. " In adult consciousness, the idea of intention, of end or aim, is the essential factor in classifying our memories. If we were simply conscious of each action by itself, and did not group the different actions in reference to different separate aims, how difficult our memory would be. On the other hand, if the idea of an aim is given, our different actions become a series of steps which arrange themselves in relation to the end desired in a way which would satisfy Aristotle or Leibnitz." [1] He then goes on to quote the example of his voyage to America, and shows that the thread of purpose which

---

[1] *Genèse de l'idée de temps*, p. 36.

unites his actions will also guide his memories of those actions. The truth of this is obvious if we contrast the difficulty of ordering the memories of a day passed in disconnected occupations conducted without a settled plan with those of one in which we have followed a definite line of action ; or, in the example given above, if we contrast the calculations necessary to determine the order of the different disconnected occupations with the simplicity of following out the course of the actions involved in one of them.

It is not only purpose or cause and effect which will act as a principle of time order ; any apprehended relation between the different events will serve to organize them into a series. A very simple experiment will show the effect of this in material which is easily remembered. Coloured papers were used of the size of post cards. Four of these were held up in succession for about 5 seconds each. Immediately after the last had been shown a lecture was begun. After an interval of 3 days the students were asked to write out the colours in the order in which they had been shown. The colours in the first series shown were white, yellow, orange, red : 44 students did the test, and there were 2 incorrect reproductions or 4·5%. The colours in the second series were orange, green, white, blue ; 36 students did the test and there were 13% errors. In the first series it was easy to apprehend the principle of the arrangement, in the second no such obvious principle existed. The consequence is that, in spite of the practice gained from the former test and the greater knowledge of what was expected, there was nearly three times the percentage of errors in the second that there was in the first.

Country dances supply a further illustration of this principle ; it is difficult to learn the order of the figures in a dance, since there seems to be no reason for that order, and the order is rapidly forgotten if practice is interrupted, yet the figures themselves are quite easy to learn and remember.

When we are dealing with events which cannot easily be arranged by means of any internal connexion we employ some kind of " dating ". In the case of a morning filled by disconnected activities we generally use times as the points from which to calculate. We determine some event as occurring at a certain time and then, by a more or less elaborate process of reasoning, relate other events to it. If the events are more remote, or cover a longer period, we employ dates in cases where precision is possible ; or if the date cannot be determined, we refer the event to some epoch :—" That was when I was quite young " ; or " when I was at school " ; or " it must have been in the summer of the year that So-and-so came back to England ".

Without some aids of this sort it seems impossible to arrange the events of past years in a series with any accuracy, and these aids depend on accumulated knowledge and experience which is worked up into a system to which events are related. These systems may be of various kinds. Some are concrete, others are of an abstract kind and are denoted by conventional time marks—hour, month, or year dates. This latter type is only possible after the whole process necessary for the development of the calendar has been gone through, and the knowledge of a calendar does not ensure its use. Even among educated adults there are great differences in the readiness with which dates are used. Some people will say without hesitation, " I first learned to punt in 1908." Others wishing to " date " a similar fact will say, " I learned to punt the year I first came to Oxford. I was living at Brighton. It must be about 10 years ago now."

The first method is undoubtedly the more convenient, though it may not be the more exact. The date gives a short cut, removes the need of irrelevant associations, and is more directly comprehensible by others. The more frequently we go over our store of memories and review them with the intention of communicating or organizing them, the more likely we are to attach dates to them and thus save ourselves time when we wish to refer to them again.

Guyau claims that all this ordering of time is not really temporal but spatial. " It is generally noticed how greatly this mechanism (arrangement in time) resembles that by which we localize points in space. There, too, we have points of reference, short cuts, and well known distances which we use as units of measurement. But M. Ribot could have added that there was more than an analogy : there is identity. In truth, when we localize an event in time, we attach our points of reference to space, and our short cuts, so well described by MM. Taine and Ribot, are in reality spatial short cuts, representations of mental pictures, with the distances vaguely imagined which receive definiteness by means of number. . . . Our representation even of time itself, our image of time, is in a spatial form." [1]

[1] *Genèse de l'idée de temps*, p. 69.

In many cases this is true. Time for some people is a line along which, at definite intervals, events are placed. This manner of representation is extremely common. The savage who tells off years on a notched stick uses a spatial form by which to represent time, the modern historian who represents periods on a time-chart does exactly the same ; and this use of space to represent time has become traditional in popular thought. On the other hand, there seems no need to believe that this method of representation is universal or that " we can only represent the past as a perspective behind us, and the future stretching from the present as a perspective in front of us. The primitive representation of time for an animal and a child must be a simple line of images more or less obliterated ".[1]

Such a line of time is a comparatively late development. It has been the whole aim of this chapter to prove that it involves reasoning and conscious arrangement, and in the form described by Guyau it also necessitates visual imagery as the normal mode of thought about time. To see time or our lives stretching as a perspective before and behind us we must visualize with a considerable degree of vividness. This visualization is implied in the French words used (figures . . . tableaux visibles . . . representer), and for a visualizer it is hard to think of any other method of arranging time which would be equally convenient. But it is quite possible to have a conception of time without such visualization. An audile might equally well, if encouraged, represent periods of time to himself as notes

[1] Guyau, op. cit., p. 70.

of varying duration, and a person possessed of motor imagery need not be devoid of a time scheme even though he habitually uses neither visual nor auditory imagery to express it.

The possibility of other forms of time representation does not, however, prevent the visual from being the most generally convenient. When dealing with times, especially those beyond our own experience, e.g. historical time, some form of representation is necessary to counteract the illusion due to differing amounts of knowledge of the different periods. A time scheme or chart based on notes of different lengths, or occurring at different intervals, might serve the purpose very well ; but it has not the permanence of a chart based on space. Nor would it, probably, be so easy to remember even by the non-visualizers. A chart hung on the wall can be referred to again and again, and looked at idly in spare moments ; a sound rhythm must be specially repeated each time it is required, and the smaller number of presentations would decrease the permanence of the knowledge gained from it. It seems better, therefore, to accept the convenience of a spatial representation of time, even though it is not, as Guyau suggests, the only possible one, nor one innately given.

CHAPTER VIII

THE NATURE OF TIME

I HAVE sketched in earlier chapters various stages in the development of the time-concept, and have indicated some of its more important constituents. In this chapter the aim is to show that time *is* a concept, and that this concept is constructed by each individual under the influence of the society in which he lives.

To say that time is a concept is not to deny that it has a certain experiential basis, and in discussing this we shall go back to the question of the first chapter, the nature of time ; only, now, that question will be discussed from a psychological standpoint.

Time as experienced possesses two main elements, and there are two others which are of less importance.

Our experience is made up of a succession of mental states, and these states must be understood to include the whole complex of our awareness at any moment ; our thoughts, our bodily sensations, and the appearances of the external world. As experienced, a moment of time is simply one of these states. We label these states in reference to some conventional time scheme, e.g. 5 o'clock on last Monday afternoon, but the *meaning* to which this phrase refers is the experience which occurred at that moment. The natural way in which to refer to a past time is " when you did so-and-so ", thus directly recalling the past state. The label from conventional time is generally preferred as being quicker and more universal in meaning, but it only acquires this universality by meaning a different thing to each person.

In consequence of this, the shortest space of time that can be directly apprehended is the shortest time in which we can experience a mental content. This is far from being as small as the amount of time one can imagine or even measure. Hence the difficulties over the divisibility of time.

The second main element in the time experience is that such states of consciousness do not come to us disconnected, but as filling a place in a time scheme. Each experience of our own is apprehended as adding a new bit on to our past. We carry our past about with us, and as an author adds a page or so to the growing pile of his manuscript, so each evening we go to bed with a certain amount added to our past life, and wake up next morning consciously older by so much. This consciousness of the " time setting " of each event is a part of our experience, it is not something which we add on to an unfixed event. It is closely comparable to the scheme of space to which we refer our movements, and is subject to perturbations in the same way. On waking from sleep it is no uncommon thing to lie for a while spatially lost, wondering where one is and unable perhaps even to determine the relation of the bed to the rest of the room ; so, too, one may for similar short periods be " lost " in time. A curious example of this is on record, where a married woman waking from sleep was not only disoriented in time but actually fitted her present experience on to the wrong part of her history.

She reports [1] : "One night in December I awoke from a dreamless sleep, wide awake, and yet to my own consciousness the little girl of years ago, in my own room in the old home. My sister had gone away (her sister used to sit with her till she fell asleep), I was alone in the darkness. I sat up in bed, and called with all my voice, ' Jessie, Jessie ' —my sister's name. This aroused my husband, who spoke to me. I seemed to come gradually to a realization of my surroundings, and with difficulty adjusted myself to the present. In that moment I seemed to live again in the childhood days and home. For days after this strange impression was with me, and I could recall many little incidents and scenes of child-life that I had entirely forgotten."

From this individual time scheme, most people pass to a universal one, and, in so passing, they leave experience behind. Time, as we apprehend it, does include a reference to our own past history ; it does not include a reference to a world scheme. Yet this extension is so easily and universally made that the world has come to be regarded as an individual, and is spoken of as having had its " youth " and sometimes is assumed to have now reached at least " middle-age ", if not its " decline ". It follows from this assumption of a world time scheme that events are not fixed in a certain order for us only, but also for the world and hence for other people ; and we arrive at once at Universal Time. Now this time cannot be the unreliable time experience of individuals, it must be invariable ; and thus we get Newtonian Time, measured by some imaginedly

<hr>

[1] Quoted in *Occult Review*, May, 1922, p. 262.

perfect timepiece ticking with the heart-beats of the universe.

All the same this supposition of Universal Time has a certain psychological foundation. It is an observed fact that we can co-operate with other individuals in a way that depends on a common time, and we do observe apparently regular changes, or at least *changes* in the things about us. The world is not just the same on Tuesday as it was on Monday ; and, therefore, if there is change, there is at least the possibility of world time, and this world time should be one dimensional.

These facts, however, are not enough to support the superstructure of world time. Co-operation is based strictly on conventional time (when it is not due to *perceived* simultaneity or immediate succession), and could be carried on even if each individual kept, for his own purposes, " an individual time." [1]

In the second case it is true that we perceive external objects and that these objects change and that, in so far as we are in touch with them, time is not our own but common. We are not, however, always in touch with them. We are not in touch with them in dreams, we are not in touch with them to any important extent during much of our ordinary waking life, and even when we are so in touch the perception of them forms only a small part of our mental content. In so far as we are free from them our time may be our own ; if we cut ourselves off from them completely, time may be entirely our own. In

[1] For this and similar matter, see May Sinclair's *Uncanny Stories*, p. 225 sqq.

cases of hysteria we can sometimes actually see this happen. Pierre Janet [1] gives the case of a girl, Irène, whose mother had died under particularly distressing circumstances. Irène had nursed her. After her mother's death Irène appeared to forget all about it, but was subject to crises in which she lived over again all the events of the time, performed the same actions, appeared to see her mother lying on the bed, and showed the same emotions. Irène on these occasions was cut off from the world, and living in a dream world of her own. In consequence she was free of time, and, in re-experiencing past events, was setting herself back in time ; since for individuals, as has been said, time *is* only the complex of consciousness at any instant.

Irène's time was set back, but, once set at a certain point, the events unrolled in their previous order. Thus far they were conditioned by external events, though the events were in the past. There is no intrinsic reason, however, why time should not be strictly reversible, and unroll backwards as it does in the dream already quoted, or as do our memories of dreams, and as in fact it did seem to do partially in some cases of regression in shell-shock patients. The reason it does not do this more often is probably that we have formed a prejudice in favour of the cause preceding what we regard as its effect. It is our accumulated knowledge of external events which keeps time in its usual order.

This view of time is essentially different from that which regards it as a fourth dimension of space-time, though

[1] *Major Symptoms of Hysteria*, p. 37.

that view in the hands of the relativists admits of individual times. On the view put forward, a moment of time is not a something which, though it may be different with different people, yet has consequences which may be discernible to others ; it is simply a state of mind peculiar,[1] as all states of mind are, to the experiencer. The materialistic view of time gives us such phantasies as Wells' " Time Machine " and De La Mare's poor " Jim Jay ".[2] In both of these cases disturbance of the normal movement in time involved disappearance from others. Wells' hero went too fast; Jim Jay " got stuck in yesterday ", but he also was lost to his friends in spite of all their best efforts to save him. Movement in a purely mental time need have no such effects. A person sleeping quietly in bed by your side may be a hundred years away in her dreams, as she may be a thousand miles, and you none the wiser, and in no way disturbed in your enjoyment of your own present space and time. There is then no intrinsic difficulty in movement in time, the only danger is that you may be counted insane by the unenlightened if the movement involves a too complete detachment from external objects.

The same attempt to make time quasi-material is at the bottom of the discussions of the configuration of space-time.[3] The question whether space-time is elliptical, hyperbolic, or euclidian, may be mathematically important, but the discussion has little psychological reality. We are told that if time were elliptical we should get a return

<hr>

[1] For the moment I waive telepathy.
[2] In *Peacock Pie*.
[3] Broad, *Scientific Thought*.

to the same point, something like the *magnus annus* of the ancients. We do sometimes get it in a small way; we could have it on a larger scale without any great disturbance. If it were hyperbolic, the specious present of beings on different time-lines would vary. There is every reason to believe that they do. It has been pointed out, by James and Du Prel, that it is impossible to believe that a gnat, a man, and a tortoise all have the same rate of experience, and if a different rate, surely they may have a different extent of specious present. The third alternative, euclidian time, allows time to pass equally for all. This is the most unlikely, psychologically, of all the alternatives; and yet it is the one that receives the most mathematical favour.

In fact time, for psychology, can have no structure. It is not of the order of things which possess " structure ". It varies from individual to individual, and in the same individual, and may assume on occasion either of the three forms. Which it actually does take on any occasion is an entertaining speculation, but an idle one.

There is evident in much modern literature a craving to " get out of time " and to achieve a timeless state akin to that spoken of in the writings of mystics, both eastern and western. In these states the mind ceases to be conscious of time because it has entered a higher sphere in which time is not; a sphere characterized by a " clear quiet ",[1] or an all pervading rapture. In the " Fioretti " we read again and again of St. Francis and his brethren being rapt up to God and losing all sense of time. Yeats

---

[1] Yeats, *Essays : Per Amica Silentia Lunae.*

writes [1] of the moment " when all sequence comes to an end, time comes to an end, and the soul puts on the rhythmic or spiritual or luminous body, and contemplates all the events of its memory and every possible impulse in an eternal possession of itself in one single moment ".

The cause of this state is best suggested by Yeats. It is attained when " all *sequence* comes to an end ". There is no means of judging time, since there is only one event ; and, moreover, as has been said above, to estimate time a certain division of attention is necessary, and here there is no division.

This concentration of thought upon a single idea does not, however, mean that the period lacks extension. Because one cannot estimate the duration of a period, that does not mean that it is felt to have *no* duration. In discussing the nature of the experience of duration it was said that we could distinguish an extensity of experience which was different from perceived change. These states of " concentration " show the character of extensity, although they do not contain changes which would allow them to be measured.

This condition of timelessness is frequently assumed to be so perfect that it is predicated of God or the " Absolute ", which broods for ever over the unchanging thought of its own perfection. It is also predicated of the subconscious, thus bringing that disreputable concept into relation with the divine. But the reasons for the attribution of timelessness must be different in the two cases. The Absolute is timeless, because it is impossible

[1] Op. cit.

for it to change, and therefore one aspect of time experience is cut off; the subconscious, on the other hand, knows not time, apparently because its sheltered existence has not brought it into contact with the world.

Time that is felt to be irksome is the time which is conditioned by our interaction with external objects. As has been said in discussing time in dreams, our rate of thought is frequently conditioned by our rate of actions, and our servitude to time is measured by the closeness of our mental connexion with external objects and even with our own body. The subconscious is not thus bound down to reality, its activities are determined by other principles, and work by other laws than those of matter. It is, therefore, assumed to be free from time. If the mystic state of concentration is connected with the activity of the subconscious, it can, as can consciousness, be free from some aspects of time; but if dreams are also manifestations of the subconscious, and if we remember dreams at all in the way in which they are experienced, then it is not free from others. It is possible to argue that in remembering a dream we introduce the category of time from our waking experience. This may be true; but if so, why do we not always introduce that type of time experience with which we are familiar. The very variability of the time experience in dreams suggests that we do remember what is actually experienced, and that this experience is different from, and perhaps inferior to, the normal one which we have developed through our contact with the world about us.

Time is then part of our adaptation to our environment; and yet most men crave to be free of it, at least to some extent. It is indeed possible to gain this freedom, but at the price of cutting one's self off from external objects, and thus from much of the society of mankind and its advantages. It may even lead to the person who practises such detachment being thought mad, for he must often need to arrange his own individual space and its filling, as well as his own time. A compromise is, however, possible ; a certain limited freedom from time can be achieved without a complete severance of our connexion with external objects. A mind supplied with stories of the past and dreams of the future has a certain freedom. Supposing the affairs of everyday do not press too heavily on it, it can slip away for many hours and walk with poets long dead in the green dusk of a twilight wood, or pass to the calm unchanging regions of speculation where the roar of the passing centuries dies as a whisper on the air.

INDEX